NCER AND EMOTION

# CANCER AND EMOTION

## Psychological Preludes and Reactions to Cancer

Jennifer Hughes
*Senior Research Fellow
Department of Psychiatry
University of Southampton*

*A Wiley Medical Publication*

**JOHN WILEY & SONS**
Chichester · New York · Brisbane · Toronto · Singapore

Copyright © 1987 by John Wiley & Sons Ltd.

All rights reserved.

No part of this book may be reproduced by any means, or transmitted, or translated into a machine language without the written permission of the publisher.

*Library of Congress Cataloging in Publication Data:*
Hughes, Jennifer
Cancer and emotion.

(A Wiley medical publication)
Bibliography: p
Includes index.
1. Cancer—Psychological aspects. 2. Emotions.
3. Cancer—Psychosomatic aspects
I. Title. II. Series. (DNLM: 1. Emotions. 2. Neoplasms—etiology.
3. Neoplasms—psychology.   QZ 200 H893c
RC262.H834    1987    616.99'4'0019    86-19043

ISBN 0 471 91187 9

*British Library Cataloguing in Publication Data:*
Hughes, Jennifer
Cancer and emotion.
1. Cancer – Psychological aspects
I. Title
616.99'4'0019    RC262

ISBN 0 471 91187 9

Printed and bound in Great Britain.

# Contents

Preface .................................................................. vi

## PART I: PSYCHOLOGICAL PRELUDES TO CANCER

1. Introduction: Studying the Role of Psychological Factors in Cancer Causation ............................... 3
2. Can Stressful Experiences Contribute to Cancer Development? ........................................... 9
3. Can Depression Herald the Onset of Cancer? ......... 19
4. Is there a Cancer-Prone Personality? ..................... 24
5. Behaviour Patterns which Predispose to Cancer ...... 30
6. Cancer Screening ............................................... 32
7. Delay in Reporting Cancer Symptoms .................... 35
8. False Alarms, Hypochondriasis and Cancer Phobia . 40
9. Reactions to a Suspected Diagnosis of Cancer ........ 43

## PART II: LIVING WITH CANCER AND ITS TREATMENT

1. Introduction ...................................................... 51
2. Surgery ............................................................ 53
3. Radiotherapy .................................................... 60
4. Chemotherapy ................................................... 64
5. Attitudes and Coping Styles ................................. 70
6. Doctor-Patient Communication ............................ 76
7. Depression in Cancer Patients .............................. 82
8. Counselling ...................................................... 94
9. The Relatives .................................................... 99

## PART III: THE FINAL OUTCOME – DEATH OR LONG-TERM SURVIVAL

1. Terminal Cancer and its Aftermath ...................... 107
2. Long-term Survival ........................................... 119
3. Can Psychological Factors Affect Cancer Prognosis? ....................................................... 121

Appendix: Breast Cancer – Patients' Own Accounts ... 129

Glossary of Medical Terms used in Text ................... 142

References ............................................................ 147

Index ................................................................... 153

# Preface

Relationships between cancer and emotion are attracting increasing interest, but the voluminous scientific literature is confusing even for experts, and media presentations for the general public often give a distorted picture. In writing this book my aim was to present a balanced introductory account in non-technical language suitable for cancer patients themselves, their families, those who care for them professionally, and interested general readers.

About one person in three in the Western world will develop some form of cancer during his or her lifetime. Although cancer is so common, and although at least one-third of all cases can now be cured, it is often regarded with almost superstitious dread, and widely considered to be the most terrible of all diseases. This reputation rests on the false assumption that cancer inevitably leads to pain, disablement, disfigurement and eventually death. When I began my medical career in 1970, many doctors of the older generation never revealed a diagnosis of cancer to their patients, because they believed the knowledge would cause so much distress. This attitude is unusual today in the mid-1980s, now that honesty and skill in 'doctor-patient communication' receive greater emphasis in medical education, and information about cancer is widely available to the general public via television and radio programmes, newspapers and magazines. But despite more widespread knowledge and greater open discussion about cancer, and despite the improvements in techniques of diagnosis and treatment which enable many cases to be cured, cancer still carries a stigma.

The emotions which most people associate with cancer, then, are unpleasant ones; anxiety, depression, perhaps anger, puzzlement, or guilt. Many patients with cancer, and their relatives too, do indeed experience great emotional distress, but this need not always be so. Mood disturbances and distorted attitudes, if recognized and understood, can often be changed for the better. One purpose of this book is therefore to draw attention to the ways in which certain emotional states can increase cancer patients' suffering, influence their behaviour so as to impede successful treatment of their illness, and damage their relationships with others. I also hope to demonstrate, however, that cancer patients are not necessarily unhappy or depressed, and that personal experience of cancer can have positive consequences. Many cancer patients not only succeed in adapting to their illness, but even find their emotional life enhanced through an increased strength of character and closer personal relationships.

A rather different function of the book is to examine the evidence that psychological factors, like personality type, attitude, and experience of stressful events, help to determine who develops cancer, or whether a patient can be cured of the disease. The medical establishment has traditionally ignored such theories, whereas many cancer patients and 'alternative practitioners' are ready to embrace them with uncritical wholehearted acceptance. Both extreme attitudes can be destructive. I have tried to put the present state of knowledge in this field into perspective.

How having cancer affects the emotions, and how emotional factors may influence cancer growth, could be considered two quite separate topics. Rather than dealing with them in two separate halves of the book, however, I found a more logical and readable result was obtained by taking the cancer process chronologically. Part I therefore deals with the development of cancer and the events leading up to diagnosis; Part II with the psychological effects of subsequent treatment and follow-up; and Part III with the eventual outcome, whether this is recovery or death. Readers who do not wish to follow this sequence should find each individual chapter is self-contained. Technical terms are defined in the Glossary.

An attempt to cover a large, complicated, and controversial subject in one short volume inevitably results in some omissions and oversimplifications. I have only described a selection of the many relevant published studies, for a comprehensive review of the literature would have been beyond the scope of the book, but references to original publications are given for readers who require more detail. Wherever possible I have included case histories and quotations from patients to illustrate the points made in the text, sometimes with minor alterations to preserve confidentiality. Most of these real-life examples come from the interviews I carried out (Hughes 1982: Hughes 1985a, 1985b: Hughes & Lee 1987) during research studies about depression among patients with cancer of the lung and breast. The principles they illustrate are applicable to many other common forms of cancer in adults. Some of my research patients from the breast cancer series have written accounts of their illness in their own words for inclusion in this book. These vivid personal descriptions of what it is like to have cancer form the Appendix.

# Acknowledgements

I should like to thank all the patients who took part in research interviews or contributed written material: those medical and surgical colleagues who collaborated with me, especially Roger Buchanan for commenting on the manuscript; the Mental Health Foundation and the Medical Research Council for financial support; Deborah Lee, who carried out the interviews with patients in the continuing-care unit; Jane Dalton, for her extensive secretarial help: and my husband, Brian Barraclough, for his advice and support.

# PART I: PSYCHOLOGICAL PRELUDES TO CANCER

# 1. Introduction: Studying the Role of Psychological Factors in Cancer Causation

**CANCER AND ITS CAUSES**

For readers without a medical background, I will begin with a very brief account of the nature of cancer, and introduce some of the technical terms which will appear frequently in the text. Readers wanting more information about the physical aspects of cancer are referred to the book by Williams (1983) or the review article by Cairns (1985).

The word cancer includes a group of diseases all characterized by abnormal and excessive cell division. 'Malignant disease' is an alternative term. Over 100 individual types of cancer exist, being distinguished by the type of cell they consist of (histological type), and the part of the body where they begin (primary site). As there is a wide variation between the different types of cancer as regards the factors which cause them, the age and sex group in which they occur, how quickly they grow and how successfully they can be treated, it can be misleading to consider cancer as a single condition.

The commonest histological type of cancer is 'carcinoma', a cancer arising from the epithelial tissue which lines body surfaces, including internal ones like the digestive tract. 'Adenocarcinoma' and 'squamous cell carcinoma' are its main subtypes. Rarer histological forms of cancer are 'sarcoma', which arises from connective tissue structures like muscle or bone; 'leukaemia', which originates 'in the bone marrow and affects the blood; and 'lymphoma', which originates in lymphoid tissue. The commonest primary sites for cancer among adults in Britain are the lung, breast, bowel, uterus (including the body of the womb and the cervix), and prostate.

Most cancers begin by producing a 'primary growth' (tumour) in the tissue of origin. Unless successful treatment is given at this stage, cancer cells spread, via the bloodstream and lymphatic system, to other parts of the body, giving rise to secondary tumour deposits or 'metastases'.

About one person in three develops cancer. Many cases can be cured, so about one in five dies from the disease. Most cancer sufferers are middle-aged or elderly, but certain kinds of cancer affect children and young adults and are an important cause of death for these age groups.

Cancer probably does not have any one single cause, but a 'multifactorial aetiology', that is, several factors need to operate together in the same person to bring about the disease. Exposure to a number of environmental factors increases the risk of cancer developing. These 'carcinogenic agents' include cigarette smoke, certain industrial chemicals, dietary substances, radiation, and viruses. Inherited (genetic) differences in susceptibility to cancer exist.

According to present knowledge, the physical factors listed above only provide a partial explanation for why cancer develops in some people and not others. As in the case of any disease for which no single physical cause has been discovered, psychologically-minded people have long believed that cancer is the result of some emotional imbalance within the individual. Since laboratory evidence that psychological factors contribute to the strength of the body's 'immune defences' has been demonstrated, theories concerned with psychological contributions to cancer growth must be taken seriously (Editorial 1979, 1985).

How much clinical importance should be attached to factors like personality type, and experience of stressful events, as risk factors for cancer is yet to be determined. There is certainly no stereotyped psychological profile that can be applied to the cancer patient, as illustrated by the contrast between these three women who were all diagnosed as having breast cancer in their late thirties.

1. *An unmarried librarian had been living alone in the same house, with the same job, for many years. She was a reserved, placid, conscientious person who was normally content with her life, but she had been promoted to a position of increased responsibility the previous year and had found this beyond her capabilities. She developed mild insomnia, occasional weepiness, and feelings of inferiority, and asked to go back to her previous post; after being allowed to do so, her psychological symptoms recovered. Apart from this episode, which she regarded as relatively minor, she had not had any notable problems in her life since the death of her mother 20 years earlier. When she found a lump in her breast she consulted her doctor promptly, but denied feeling much concern.*

2. *A housewife and part-time teacher, who lived with her husband and two teenage children, was active and sociable but rather 'highly strung' and suffered from migraine. Five years earlier her mother had been treated for a lymphoma and this had worried her very much at the time, but the treatment had been a success. She had had no other problems since then, and considered her life happy and fulfilling. Discovery of a breast lump caused her great anxiety.*

3. *A housewife and part-time beautician, living with her husband and two young children, had once been extravert and cheerful, but had felt depressed and lethargic for at least a year before she found a lump in her breast. Three years previously, her husband had been treated for cancer and she was constantly worried he might relapse. Since then, her mother and several acquaintances had died from cancer of various types, and her*

*reaction had been one of anger, bitterness, and hatred of the doctors who had failed to save their lives.*

## SOME PROBLEMS OF STUDYING POSSIBLE PSYCHOLOGICAL CAUSES OF CANCER

1. Cancers of different types may have different causes. They should therefore be studied separately.

2. The factors responsible for the onset of a cancer (initiating factors) may be different from those responsible for subsequent growth of that cancer (promoting factors). Initiating and promoting factors should be studied separately, if possible.

3. A mixture of factors acting together is almost certainly concerned in cancer growth. Factors other than the one under study should therefore be controlled for when designing and analysing research.

4. Animal experiments, which are so widely used in investigating physical causes of cancer, have little relevance to psychological causes. Personality, mood, attitudes, and 'stress' in animals can only be measured in a very crude fashion which probably bears little relation to human experience.

5. Even in humans, there is no generally accepted way of defining and measuring most psychological variables exactly. Results of different studies can therefore vary according to the method chosen. For example, people who tend to conceal their emotions and strive to present a socially acceptable front (as it is claimed cancer patients are prone to do) may not score as 'depressed' on a self-rating questionnaire even if they do have depressive symptoms; a study including personal interviews instead of questionnaires is more likely to elicit their true state of mind.

6. Cause and effect are often impossible to disentangle, as discussed below under 'retrospective studies'.

## PROSPECTIVE AND RETROSPECTIVE STUDIES

Research studies can be broadly divided into those with prospective and retrospective designs. In general, prospective ones are scientifically sounder but retrospective ones are easier to carry out.

### Prospective Studies

Groups of people, who are apparently free from cancer when they enter the study, are given psychological assessments at the beginning, and then followed up to see whether the results of these assessments help to predict which of them have developed cancer by the end. The practical problem is that such studies are only successful if they are done on a massive scale.

Thousands of people need to be included to make sure that a reasonable number of them will develop cancer during the duration of the study. This duration needs to be long, preferably 10 or 20 years, since there is an interval of this order (the 'latent period') between the true onset of a cancer, and the time it first causes symptoms or can be detected by tests. Because of these daunting requirements, prospective studies based on personal interviews are seldom carried out on this topic. A quicker alternative is using documentary evidence collected some years earlier for another purpose, for example medical case records or census data.

### Retrospective Studies

Patients who already have cancer are compared with cancer-free 'control' subjects. In many studies of this kind, patients are assessed when they first present to hospital with suspected cancer, but before having tests to prove or disprove the diagnosis. Patients in whom cancer is subsequently confirmed are then compared with those who turn out not to have the disease. There are several pitfalls in interpreting the results of retrospective studies:

1. The presence of the cancer may influence patients' psychological state, either because
(a) the physical effects of the disease (for example brain metastases) are affecting them
(b) they know or suspect they have this serious disease.

2. Sick people often try to explain the onset of their illness in terms of 'stress' and this can lead them to exaggerate the number or severity of their problems without meaning to do so.

3. The 'control' patients, though they do not have cancer, have sought medical attention for other reasons. Such patients may
(a) be suffering from other physical diseases, which might cause or be caused by psychological factors just as cancer might;
(b) have consulted their doctors because they have unrecognized psychological disturbances which produce physical symptoms or hypochondriacal ideas.

4. The latent period for cancer cannot be measured in any individual, so it is impossible to know whether any past 'life events' or depressive episodes occurred before or after the onset of the disease.

The problems in designing research studies which will produce valid information about psychological precursors of cancer are clearly formidable, and will be repeatedly illustrated by the studies quoted in later sections.

# 2. Can Stressful Experiences Contribute to Cancer Development?

The idea that the loss of a close relationship, or other stressful 'life event', can bring about a serious physical illness such as cancer appeals to a great many patients, and seems to fit with their own experiences. The medical establishment has taken little notice of this idea until fairly recently, but there is now ample evidence from laboratory research to show that events like bereavement are often followed by changes in the body's hormone balance and immune defences (Editorial, 1985). Such changes might, in theory, encourage the growth of cancer in predisposed people. As yet, however, studies of cancer patients have failed to establish one way or the other whether this is really an important effect in clinical terms. The topic is a difficult one to research (Paykel and Rao, 1984), and I will start by pointing out some of the difficulties before going on to describe the results of some published studies.

## RESEARCH PROBLEMS

1. Many types of cancer have started to grow many years before they first cause any symptoms, and there is no way of telling how long this latent period has been for any individual patient. So if a newly diagnosed cancer patient recalls an important 'life event' a few years back, it is impossible to know whether this took place before or after the cancer began to develop. Certain life events might even have been brought about in the first place because an occult cancer was changing the patient's behaviour.

Most studies have not taken account of cancer's long latent

period and have only considered periods of five years, or less, before the patient presents for treatment. Life events during such periods might conceivably have caused the cancer to grow more quickly, but could not have been responsible for starting off the disease.

2. Measuring life events and their impact is far from simple. Consider, for example, one common event, the death of a mother. The impact of this event on the child might vary from trivial to catastrophic, depending on many factors including the ages of both mother and child, how often they saw one another and how close the relationship was, and whether the death was sudden or followed a long illness.

The 'objective' impact of the event — how important or unpleasant it would seem to be to the average observer when all the circumstances are taken into account — may be different from the 'subjective' impact, that is how the person concerned actually perceives the event. Subjective impact might be more important than objective impact when considering whether life events influence susceptibility to cancer. One could speculate that people who react with depression, guilt or despair after adverse life events would become more vulnerable to illness, whereas people who take similar events as a challenge, or as an opportunity for personal growth, might have their defences against disease strengthened!

Some methods of measuring life events always give the same numerical score to a defined event like 'death of mother', this score being based on the impact of this event for the average member of a large population. Other methods, more ambitious and time-consuming, consider every individual event in its unique context before rating its impact (for example Brown and Harris, 1978).

Much life event research is done on the assumption that memory is accurate, but this is not always so. Even for big events like births, deaths, marriages, and divorces, people soon forget which year they occurred, let alone how they felt about the event at the time. If patients who are under investigation for suspected cancer are being interviewed about past life events, they may unwittingly exaggerate their unpleasantness, either because they want to find a reason for their illness ('effort after meaning'), or because they are unhappy about their current circumstances.

3. Is it necessary to use a comparison (control) group to find out whether cancer patients have more stressful events in their lives than anyone else? Losses like parents' deaths occur in almost everyone's experience, and one could argue that even if cancer patients do not have any more life events than anyone else, they may react to them differently, or that the average ration of events is sufficient to cause cancer in predisposed people.

In most studies it has been thought necessary to use a comparison group, and the most convenient one in retrospective studies consists of patients who are referred to hospital with suspected cancer but turn out not to have this condition. Such patients, however, usually have other types of illness, which might equally well have been brought about by 'stress'. A comparison group from the general population would be better in some ways, but few of the studies which have tried to use this kind have managed to achieve cooperation from a satisfactory proportion of people.

Whatever comparison group is chosen, its members should be matched with the cancer group for age and sex, which influence the frequency of many life events: for example, the chances of being widowed are greater for a 60-year-old woman than for either a 50-year-old woman or a 60-year-old man.

In the remainder of this section I will summarize some studies which have sought an association between life event experience and cancer. The reader should note that studies of the kind described here can never prove the presence of a direct cause-and-effect relationship, they can only seek statistical associations which suggest a true link.

## A PROSPECTIVE RECORDS STUDY

Data about widowhood from the 1971 census of England and Wales was examined in relation to national cancer registrations and deaths for the next ten years (Jones *et al.*, 1984). Widowed people were found to develop cancer slightly more often than the rest of the population, but the small size of the excess suggested that, even if there is a direct cause-and-effect relationship between widowhood and cancer, it is not a very important one.

The results of this study must be valid, since it was based on accurate data about a single major life event from thousands of people. Even though it was unable to consider the kind of detailed information obtainable through direct interviews, such as the subjects' reactions to being widowed and the degree of social support available to them afterwards, it provides strong evidence against the theory that bereavement is a powerful cause of cancer.

I do not know of a prospective interview study about life events and the onset of cancer (though there are some about life events in relation to the prognosis of already-diagnosed cancer, which are considered in Section III.3 of this book). Some of the many retrospective ones are described next. Designing a perfect retrospective study on this topic is almost impossible and all the studies quoted, including my own, possess methodological flaws.

## RETROSPECTIVE STUDIES

A New York psychoanalyst (Le Shan, 1966) obtained detailed life histories from 450 cancer patients, some of whom were in psychotherapy with him, and was able to identify a characteristic pattern which applied to over 70% of them but was much less common in his 'control' patients who did not have cancer. The majority of cancer patients reported that before they were about seven years old they had some experience which impaired their ability to relate to others: sometimes this was a defined event like the death of a close family member, sometimes it was less clearcut. After this they experienced inner guilt, isolation, and a sense of failure, though on the surface they coped with life quite well and grew up to be decent, conforming people. In young adulthood, they abandoned their mental isolation to form an extremely strong attachment to another person, a career or a cause, and poured all their energy into this. After a variable time they lost the object of their attachment, and although they continued to cope superficially, they suffered an inner devastation. The first symptoms of cancer supervened anything from six months to eight years later.

This study, though large and thorough, fails to fulfil several of the requirements which are desirable in research and therefore it is impossible to judge whether the findings are valid. The patients were not randomly selected, but a special subgroup who seemed in need of psychotherapy. The investigator already knew they had cancer before he carried out the assessments, and these were not gathered or analysed in a systematic manner which could easily be reproduced: the characteristic pattern is described in such flexible terms that a wide variety of life histories could be fitted into it. Nevertheless, the findings are interesting and they are of a rather subtle kind, difficult to translate into exactly measurable terms for the purpose of a rigidly designed scientific inquiry. The following study illustrates an attempt to do this.

Women about to have a breast lump biopsied were interviewed using a standard format (Muslin *et al.,* 1966). After the results of the biopsy were known, each patient found to have breast cancer was paired with a benign breast disease patient of the same age, race, marital status, and socioeconomic background. Psychiatrists who had not been told the patients' diagnoses analysed the interview material and made judgements as to whether there had been any separation from an important person during the past three years and/or before the patient was nine years old. Thirty-seven pairs were analysed, sufficient to conclude there was no difference between the cancer group and the benign group as regards the number of separations experienced. The careful methodology used in this work means the results cannot have been biased by selection of patients or by the investigators' preconceived theories. A number of similar studies on breast cancer have since been published (for example Greer and Morris, 1975; Schonfield, 1975; Priestman *et al.*, 1985) and have failed to demonstrate that breast cancer patients experience any more loss events than comparison women, usually women with benign breast disease, in periods of up to five years before their diagnosis is made. The cancers had probably been growing for considerably longer than this.

Interviews concerned with the number and severity of 'emotion-provoking events' over a whole lifetime were given to 44 men with cancer and 44 men (matched for age and social characteristics) with other diseases in a Texas hospital (Smith and Sebastian, 1976). The cancer patients reported nearly twice the total number of events, and nearly three times as many events judged 'high' in their emotional implication. The flaw in the study is that the patients were already aware of their diagnosis, although the interviewers had not been told, and those who knew they had cancer might well have been influenced by 'effort after meaning' to report more stress.

The possible role of life events in precipitating childhood cancer was examined by comparing 25 children attending a New York hospital for the treatment of malignant disease, usually leukaemia or lymphoma, with 25 children of similar age and sex who had less serious diseases (Jacobs and Charles, 1980). The children's parents filled in a life events questionnaire covering the year before diagnosis, and were interviewed about the previous two years. The children with cancer were reported to have had about twice as many events in their families as the control group, for example there had been a marital separation in 32% of cancer families but only 12% of control families, and a death in 20% of cancer families but only 4% of control ones. Again, since both groups of parents knew their child's diagnosis, 'effort after meaning' may have biased the results: items like 'death in the family', unless tightly defined to specify exactly which categories of relatives should be included, can be interpreted in varying ways.

A study on patients with chest conditions (Horne and Picard, 1979) found that 68% of lung cancer patients but only 33% of patients with non-malignant chest diseases had experienced the death of a first degree relative, or lost a job, in the five years before diagnosis. Though the patients in this study were interviewed before the diagnosis was made, the result could have been affected by the fact that the lung cancer patients were an older group. In my own study on lung cancer, I inquired about the frequency of six events (death of a spouse, death of a first-degree relative, life-threatening illness of a spouse or first-degree relative, giving up work, a child leaving home, and moving house) during the past two years for 50 lung cancer patients interviewed just before diagnosis, and for 50 age/sex matched controls from the general population. The frequency of all six events was virtually identical in both groups.

Identical twin pairs in which one twin develops cancer form ideal subjects for studies of this kind, for identical twins have the same genetic make-up and differences in their susceptibility to disease must result from environmental factors. Twenty-two such pairs were obtained through an American centre where healthy twins acted as donors of bone marrow to their co-twins suffering from leukaemia (Smith *et al.*, 1984). Life events for the three years before leukaemia was diagnosed were elicited by a standard questionnaire. The result was the opposite of what had been predicted, for the healthy twins reported more life events than the sick twins. No analysis of individual events is given and so it is not clear whether the higher scores for the healthy twins resulted from 'positive' life events like marriage or a new job, or from the 'loss' events which are postulated as being conducive to cancer.

I interviewed 140 women with undiagnosed breast lumps before they attended a hospital clinic, and asked about certain defined events during the past 15 years. Data on 37 cancer patients, and 37 age-matched patients with benign breast disease, resulted.

The analysis presented first (Table 1) is restricted to a few major events which most women would find stressful and

Table 1. 37 breast cancer patients and 37 age-matched women with benign breast disease compared on 'major loss'* before diagnosis

|  | Number of (%) of patients with one or more losses |
|---|---|
| 0-5 years ago |  |
| Cancer | 15(41%) |
| Benign | 13(35%) |
| 5-10 years ago |  |
| Cancer | 11(30%) |
| Benign | 7(19%) |
| 10-15 years ago |  |
| Cancer | 12(32%) |
| Benign | 11(30%) |
| Whole 15 years |  |
| Cancer | 29(78%) |
| Benign | 28(76%) |

Total number of 'major loss' events for whole period:
 Cancer 43
 Benign 33

*'Major loss' is defined as the death of a husband, parent or sibling, or divorce.

should be able to time with reasonable accuracy after several years had passed: death of a husband, parent, brother or sister, or divorce. Table 1 shows that the patients who turned out to have cancer did report slightly more of these major losses over the entire time span and especially 5-10 years before the interviews. But the differences are small and, of course, many other stressful events have been left out of consideration because they are so difficult to define or recall precisely. If, rather than just this restricted list of major events, anything the patient herself considered stressful is included, then 90% of all patients had had 'stress' in the five years before interview: this includes things like the death of a close friend, an unhappy marriage, caring for a chronically sick parent.

Secondly, to examine the idea that cancer patients are distinguished by their personal reaction to events, rather than the number or type of events they experience, patients' subjective reports about their reactions to whatever was happening in their lives during various time periods is given (for the 33 pairs on whom there was enough information) in Table 2.

Table 2. Subjective impact of events and stresses for 33 breast cancer patients and 33 age-matched women with benign breast disease

|  | Severe | Moderate | Mild | None |
|---|---|---|---|---|
| Year before diagnosis |  |  |  |  |
| Cancer | 6 | 13 | 3 | 11 |
| Benign | 6 | 8 | 10 | 9 |
| 1-5 years before diagnosis |  |  |  |  |
| Cancer | 8 | 8 | 2 | 15 |
| Benign | 1 | 15 | 6 | 11 |
| 5-10 years before diagnosis |  |  |  |  |
| Cancer | 5 | 6 | 1 | 21 |
| Benign | 1 | 9 | 4 | 19 |

The same number of cancer and benign patients reported severe subjective stress in the year before interview, but further back in time the cancer patients reported rather more. It would be wrong to attach too much importance to this result, for the cancer patients may have had correct suspicions about their diagnosis which coloured their memories in a darker light.

Individual case histories illustrate the marked variation in the type and timing of 'stress' before a cancer is diagnosed. The following are all from breast cancer cases.

*1. (Separated, early 40's) Three years previously her husband suddenly left home. This unexpected shock caused her severe distress and many practical problems, but despite constant anxiety she successfully strove to keep going, caring for three school-age children and frail parents and getting a job.*

*2. (Married, mid-50's) She had lived happily in the same house with her husband and son for many years. Her father had died 12 years earlier: 'the greatest upset of my life, but time heals.'*

*3. (Married, early 60's) Retirement, an enforced move of house, a mother having to enter a nursing home and a daughter needing psychiatric treatment, all in the past year. She kept calm and did not get depressed.*

*4. (Married, late 40's) She was happily married, enjoyed her job, and was looking forward to moving to a new house. There had been no real problems in her life since her father died 22 years before.*

## SUMMARY

The question of whether stressful events can contribute to causing cancer is extraordinarily difficult to investigate, and most published studies have flaws of one kind or another which make it impossible to draw definite conclusions from their results. On balance, there is little evidence that cancer patients have experienced more stressful events in their lives than other people. But it could still be true that stressful events are among the factors which encourage growth of cancer in predisposed people, and laboratory studies have shown a physical basis for such an effect.

# 3. Can Depression Herald the Onset of Cancer?

This section examines the evidence as to whether depression of mood is unusually common in patients who, though still apparently in good physical health, are shortly going to show the first signs or symptoms of cancer.

Depression and cancer are both common conditions, so they are sometimes bound to develop at about the same time in the same person purely by chance. If a greater than chance association between them does exist, one or more of three possible mechanisms could be responsible:

1. The depression could produce physiological changes permitting a latent cancer to develop more rapidly, for depression is known to be accompanied by changes in hormone balance and immune competence. This theory is closely linked with the one discussed in the previous section about stressful 'life events' initiating or promoting cancer growth, since depression is often precipitated by such events.

2. The cancer, already present although not yet recognized, could be causing complications which affect the working of the brain and so produce depression. Complications of cancer which might have this effect include cerebral metastases (secondary tumour deposits in the brain), and ectopic hormone secretion (production of chemicals which circulate in the blood stream, and might affect mood by their effect on brain cells).

3. Similar factors could be responsible for causing both depression and cancer, for example the two conditions might have a partially shared inherited tendency.

Rather than dwell on these theoretical mechanisms in any greater detail, I will describe some of the studies designed to find out whether there really is an association between depression and the early stages of cancer. Investigations on this topic are hampered by the usual methodological problems, already discussed in the two previous sections, which beset research into any psychological precursors of cancer. There is an additional difficulty that some of the symptoms of depression, like tiredness and lack of energy, loss of apppetite and weight, are also common symptoms of cancer.

## PROSPECTIVE RECORD STUDIES

Two follow-up studies on patients treated for depression in psychiatric hospitals (Kerr *et al.,* 1969; Whitlock and Siskind 1979) found an unexpectedly high rate of deaths from cancer over the next four years for middle-aged or elderly men. To investigate this finding on a larger scale, the number of cancer registrations for patients treated by the Oxford psychiatric services over the previous four years was examined (Evans *et al.,* 1974), but proved to be no greater than expected by chance.

## RETROSPECTIVE CLINICAL STUDIES

Cancer of the pancreas has a particular reputation for presenting with depression. This phenomenon was studied through interviews with 125 consecutive new surgical patients who were suspected to have some kind of intra-abdominal cancer in an American centre (Fras *et al.,* 1967). Of the 46 patients who turned out to have pancreatic cancer, 35 reported that mental symptoms like depression, loss of ambition, anxiety, and premonition of serious illness, had started before or together with their first physical symptoms. Mental symptoms were far less common for the patients in this series who turned out to have bowel cancer.

For women presenting with breast lumps (Greer and Morris 1975), a history of depression during the preceding five years was found to be as common among those who turned out to have benign breast disease as among those with cancer, that is about 35% in both groups.

In my own research series of 33 breast cancer patients questioned in detail on this topic, five reported definite depressive episodes in the year before they presented to hospital, and another eight had borderline symptoms. None had been referred to a psychiatrist. There was usually a convincing external reason for their depression in the form of a recent bereavement or other loss, or chronic social problems. A few attributed their depressed mood to recent 'flu' or to the menopause, as in the following case.

*She was in her 40's and her periods were becoming irregular. She began to feel very depressed if she was alone in the house, and would spend this time weeping and brooding over the past. The depression was worse before periods occurred. Her GP prescribed hormone replacement tablets and her mental symptoms improved. This patient had a past history of mild postnatal depression after the birth of both her children.*

The frequency of depression among these breast cancer patients before diagnosis of their physical illness is no greater than that found in research studies of women in the general population (Brown and Harris, 1978).

I interviewed 138 lung cancer patients, before their diagnosis was confirmed, about recent depressive symptoms, their duration, and apparent causes. Twenty-three (17%) gave a definite history of depression in the year before they had noticed any sign of physical illness, and if borderline cases are included the number rises to 32 (24%). Two-thirds of these depressed patients had had separate episodes of depression at an earlier stage of life, a significantly higher proportion than among the rest of the sample. The cases of depression were not concentrated among any one histological type of lung cancer. Most patients attributed their depression to family and social problems: commonly death or illness of close relatives, or loneliness and isolation since widowhood or retirement, for the group was predominantly an elderly one. The frequency of a defined list of major 'life events' in the past two years was significantly greater for the depressed members of the sample than the rest. A minority had 'endogenous' depression which did not seem to be due to social circumstances.

*1. A married man in his 70's had an attack of pneumonia. The physical symptoms of this illness cleared up, but left him feeling depressed for no apparent reason, for the first time in his life. He lost interest in his hobbies, could not concentrate on simple activities, got irritable with his wife, and had spells of weeping. This depression continued for four years. Then he developed a persistent cough and his chest X-ray demonstrated a shadow. Investigation revealed a squamous cell carcinoma of the lung.*

*2. A man of 75, with no previous history of depression, attempted to commit suicide with an overdose of his wife's sleeping pills. He was revived, and psychiatric assessment revealed a severe 'endogenous' depression. He remained depressed on and off over the next five years, though he made temporary improvements after each of several courses of ECT and antidepressant drugs. He was no longer depressed when he presented to hospital with chest pain, which proved to be due to anaplastic carcinoma of the lung.*

One other patient, a man of 70 who had been widowed eight years before, did not fulfil the research criteria for depression but made the following statement: I've never worried about anything much since my wife died. Perhaps the spirit's left. I don't care what happens — I wouldn't think of suicide, but let's say if a car happened to run into me I wouldn't take evasive action.'

The duration of depression in these lung cancer cases ranged from a few months to several years. The longest time was 20 years, in a man who had become even more depressed as his physical illness developed.

On their own, these findings suggest that depression is a common early feature of lung cancer, but very similar results were obtained from interviews with age/sex matched controls: 45 patients admitted to hospital for minor surgery and 52 people chosen at random from a GP's list. Although patients in the lung cancer group did report recent depression as slightly more frequent and more severe, the small difference can probably be explained by a tendency for sick people under investigation for cancer to be more aware of any past troubles.

Depression in the later stages of cancer will be considered in Sections I.9, II.7, and III.1.

## SUMMARY

Evidence favouring an excess frequency of depression preceding the diagnosis of cancer is rather weak. Depression is a common condition, and probably no more frequent in the very early stages of cancer than in the general population as a whole. Occasional individual cancer patients become depressed as a result of physical complications of their undiagnosed tumour, but this does not seem to be a common effect for most cancers: it may occur more often with some tumours like cancer of the pancreas. Depression in patients with very early cancer usually develops following social stress, like depression in physically healthy people, and its coexistence with the cancer is probably due to chance.

# 4. Is there a Cancer-Prone Personality?

Personality is the unique combination of emotional characteristics, or traits, which distinguish one individual from another. In theory, personality traits are stable over time, yet personality does possess flexibility, often gradually changing as a person grows older. In some people transient alterations of feeling and behaviour, probably resulting from changes in their mood or circumstances, can be so striking that they mask their 'real' personality.

Personality can be assessed by various methods, and described according to various schemes. Some of these involve allocating people to one of several personality 'types', for example the obsessional personality, the hysterical personality, depending on their most prominent characteristics. Many people do not easily fit any preconceived type. A more sensitive but more complicated approach involves measuring the degree to which each of certain personality traits, for example optimism, sensitivity, anxiety, self-confidence, are present in each person. Whatever classification system is being used, assessment should be based on some standardized measurement like a questionnaire, for assessments which simply rely on an interviewer's impression depend too much on the interviewer's own personality to be reliably compared with assessments done by someone else.

Results of studies on the personalities of cancer patients do show some consistency, one frequently reported trait being the tendency not to show much emotion, especially unpleasant emotion like anger or hostility. The explanation for this association is not known, though it seems to make intuitive sense to suppose it is due to cause and effect and that a lifetime of 'bottling up' painful emotions might eventually lead to these being expressed physically through the development of a malignant tumour. The true explanation could be quite different; for example there could be a genetic link between personality type and vulnerability to cancer. Or certain personality types might be more likely than others to choose behaviour patterns which increase risk of cancer, or less likely to heed advice on cancer prevention (Sections I.5 and I.6).

I will describe some of the studies which have sought evidence for a 'cancer-prone personality'. Many of them are retrospective, carried out when the cancer was already there even if not yet diagnosed, and one cannot discount the possibility that either the presence of the cancer, or the patient's suspicions about it, influenced the results.

## PROSPECTIVE STUDIES

A personality questionnaire called the MMPI (Dahlstrom *et al.*, 1975) was completed by 2020 male employees of a company in Chicago (Shekelle *et al.*, 1981). Men who scored highly on the depression scale of this questionnaire were twice as likely to die from cancer throughout the subsequent 17-year follow-up period as the rest of the men in the sample.

Another American study based on the MMPI obtained a dissimilar result (Dattore *et al.*, 1980). Seventy-five men being treated for cancer in a Veterans' Administration hospital were found to have obtained lower MMPI depression scores, when psychologically tested some years before, than the control group of 125 men hospitalized for other diseases. The cancer group in this study also showed greater repression of emotion, which is in keeping with the results of other work.

In a prospective study of American college students (Thomas *et al.*, 1979), self-reported lack of closeness to parents in childhood was found to be associated with development of cancer during the next 20 years.

## RETROSPECTIVE STUDIES

### Lung Cancer

Patients admitted to a chest hospital in Scotland for investigation were given a standard interview before their diagnosis was established (Kissen, 1963). The 154 men who were found to have lung cancer differed from 166 men with non-malignant conditions in their tendency to conceal emotional problems: 60% of the cancer patients in contrast to 43% of the rest usually 'bottled up feelings'. The difference was most marked for the youngest (under 54) and oldest (over 65) patients. The cancer patients also recalled less behaviour disturbance during childhood.

Early psychoanalytically-based studies described cancer patients as being rigid, resistant to change, and lacking in creativity or imaginative power. An interview regarding lifestyle, designed to explore these traits, was given to 59 patients being investigated for chest disease in an American hospital (Abse *et al.*, 1974). The differences between the 31 patients who were found to have lung cancer and the 28 who were not depended on age. For younger patients the results were in the predicted direction, for the cancer patients were reported to be excessively conscientious, to have fewer and less adequate personal and sexual relationships, to have greater marital stability (which is interpreted as showing long-suffering and social conformity rather than as a sign of happy marriage!), and recall fewer dreams.

In another American study (Horne and Picard, 1979) five items thought to have an association with cancer were rated at interview for 110 men with chest X-ray abnormalities, and the results used to predict what the diagnosis would be. These items — childhood instability, job stability, marriage stability, lack of plans for the future, and an important loss in the past five years — predicted the correct diagnosis with more than chance accuracy.

Table 3. Response to problems, and expression of anger, in lung cancer patients and general population controls

|  | Lung cancer ($n=65$) | Controls ($n=52$) |
|---|---|---|
| 1. Usual response to a problem | | |
| Talk it over | 33(51%) | 30(58%) |
| Keep it to oneself | 27(42%) | 19(37%) |
| Never has any problems | 5(8%) | 3(6%) |
| 2. Usual response when angered | | |
| Lose one's temper | 28(43%) | 21(40%) |
| Talk problem over | 10(15%) | 14(27%) |
| Say nothing | 21(32%) | 12(23%) |
| Never feels angry | 3(5%) | 0(0%) |
| Uncertain | 3(5%) | 4(8%) |

For 65 of the patients in my own study on lung cancer, and 52 age/sex matched general population controls, the interview included two questions regarding the expression of emotion. One concerned their usual way of dealing with a worrying problem: did they talk it over with another person or keep it to themselves? The other concerned their usual response when angered: did they lose their temper, try to talk the matter over, or say nothing? The result (Table 3) showed the lung cancer had a slightly greater tendency to 'bottle up' worries or anger, or deny ever experiencing them at all, but the difference between the two groups is too small to be significant.

## Cervical Cancer

Forty American women who had cervical smears suspicious of cancer were given interviews to explore their tendency towards 'hopelessness' (Schmale and Iker, 1966). The 14 who did prove to have cancer were found to show more 'hopelessness' than the rest: features contributing to a high hopelessness rating included the tendency to react to adverse events with feelings of guilt and responsibility for failure, and inability to feel pleasure or satisfaction as a result of personal accomplishment.

The women with cancer also scored more highly than the rest on the depression scale of the MMPI.

## Breast Cancer

Fifty women about to have a breast biopsy were questioned about their usual way of expressing anger (Morris *et al.*, 1981). Expression of anger was rated on a six-point scale, ranging from 'does not admit to feeling anger ever since age 21' to 'loses control in anger at least once a month in front of adults'. The 17 patients who proved to have cancer, especially those under 50, reported feeling less anger, and being less likely to express what anger they did feel, than the 33 patients with benign breast disease.

Personality assessment was not a main aim of my own studies on breast cancer, but indirect confirmation of the unaggressive nature of breast cancer patients compared to those with benign breast disease comes from one of the questions about recent life events: had they had any marked conflict with another person during the past year? Only one (3%) of 33 cancer patients answered yes to this question, in contrast to 27 (25%) of the 107 benign breast patients.

The 44 breast cancer patients in my earlier study had been asked to describe their personalities in their own words as part of the initial interview assessment. Their descriptions were, of course, quite varied, but terms like 'contented', 'cheerful', 'happy', 'calm', 'placid', and 'easygoing' were often used, and only a few patients considered themselves 'tense', 'a worrier', 'quick-tempered' or prone to depression. Nearly all the patients volunteered that they enjoyed practical activities like gardening or knitting. With few exceptions these patients were cooperative in the research interview, and most appeared emotionally composed, resigned rather than obviously anxious or depressed about the prospect of mastectomy. While I have no control group against which to evaluate these descriptive observations, they are in keeping with the typical cancer patient profile which emerges from the various research studies: pleasant, unemotional, stable, and calm.

## SUMMARY

The personality characteristic most often described in cancer patients is a reduced ability to feel or express emotion, especially hostility or anger. The differences in personality between cancer patients and other people are relatively small. Not all cancer patients possess these characteristics, and many healthy people do possess them but never develop cancer. There is no evidence that trying to change such characteristics can reduce risk of cancer, and why they should have a link with cancer is not known.

# 5. Behaviour Patterns which Predispose to Cancer

Behaviour which is under voluntary control can affect susceptibility to cancer. Cigarette smoking and its link with lung cancer is the best example, because this link is firmly established and well-publicized. Individual factors like personality, and group factors like social custom and fashion, help to determine whether people consider that smoking is an attractive pastime at all, and also whether they think the pleasure of smoking is worth the extra risk of developing cancer in the future. When the relationship between smoking and lung cancer was discovered, many young people decided never to take up smoking, and many people who already smoked managed to give up. Others carried on, for a variety of reasons:

*Conscious choice:* 'I enjoy my cigarettes. If I get lung cancer that's just too bad.'

*Insufficient willpower to overcome an addiction:* 'I've tried all sorts of ways to give up. I know it's harming my health but I just can't stop.'

*Denial:* 'I know they say some people get lung cancer, but cigarettes never did me any harm.'

*Rationalization, distorting the facts, and false logic:* 'I've known plenty of people who smoked and didn't get cancer.' 'I heard of a bloke who got lung cancer and he'd never smoked a cigarette in his life, so I don't think it's got anything to do with smoking at all.'

*Ignorance about the link:* The frequency of smoking among doctors declined faster than that in any other group of the population when the link between smoking and lung cancer was discovered. Despite the publicity many people, especially poorly-educated ones, probably failed to understand it properly.

Besides smoking, many other common aspects of modern lifestyle have been linked with cancer. Prolonged exposure to strong sunlight increases the risk of skin cancer. Lack of fibre in the diet increases the risk of bowel cancer. Promiscuity in young women increases the risk of cervical cancer. Women who do not have children, or who delay childbearing till later life, and who never breastfeed a child, have an increased risk of breast cancer. Most of these examples only involve a small increase in cancer risk, and these risks have not been widely publicized, so all but the most health-conscious section of the population are probably either unaware of them, or have decided to ignore them. Sometimes a whole group of people decide to take a calculated risk, for example when the contraceptive pill was introduced, many women and their doctors believed it might turn out to induce cancer of the breast or female sexual organs after prolonged use, but they still decided to use it because they thought the benefits of reliability and convenience outweighed any hypothetical risk to future health. So far, this decision has proved justified, for there is no solid evidence to link the 'Pill' with cancer.

There is nothing wrong with deciding to ignore warnings about minor risks to health: most activities in life carry some kind of danger, and everyone has to die of something! Obsessive efforts to avoid all the potentially carcinogenic aspects of the modern world would result in a highly restricted lifestyle which would still give no guarantee of good health. If knowledge of the facts is made widely available, people who wish to do so are free to adjust their lifestyle accordingly.

# 6. Cancer Screening

Cancer screening involves carrying out medical examinations and technical tests, for example cervical cytology (smear test) and mammography of the breasts, on apparently healthy people, in the hope of detecting cancers in a very early stage when there should be an excellent chance of cure.

The benefits of screening have not proved clear-cut. One reason is that many people in high-risk groups fail to take up opportunities to be screened. People who do accept screening are probably the same ones who would consult a doctor promptly if they did develop any symptoms suggestive of cancer. On the other hand, people prone to delay in revealing suspicious symptoms are also liable to ignore invitations to screening programmes.

## PSYCHOLOGICAL BARRIERS TO SCREENING

I will describe two studies designed to examine psychological barriers to cancer screening. One was concerned with attitudes to breast cancer screening, including the simple procedure of regular breast self-examination (BSE), among women in Edinburgh (Leathar and Roberts, 1985). A total of 136 women were recruited from the general population, divided into 12 small groups, and asked to discuss breast disease under the guidance of a psychologist. These women expressed much fear of breast cancer, but little correct knowledge about it. They knew most breast lumps are benign (non-cancerous) but tended to assume that any lump they themselves developed would be malignant (cancerous). Three attitudes which discouraged breast self-examination were identified, especially among older women: their sexual inhibitions made them consider it 'not nice'; they were ignorant of what to search for or how to to do it; or they carried it out so superficially that there was little danger of finding anything wrong. As for attending screening clinics, they had little practical knowledge about what services were available locally. They said such clinics were a good thing in theory, but for other women rather than for themselves. Reasons given for not attending included being too busy, not considering it important enough, embarrassment about having a physical examination or about showing distress in front of strangers if an abnormality was found, and wasting staff time if there was no abnormality. The authors conclude that emotional barriers, rather than simple ignorance, impede compliance with screening programmes, and suggest that individual counselling is needed to overcome these, since mass media presentations may well increase anxiety. Such recommendations are easier to make than to put into practice.

Bowel cancer screening was the subject of another study (Box *et al.*, 1984). Bowel cancer can be detected early by a self-administered chemical test for the presence of small amounts of blood in the faeces. Patients over 40 who were registered with one of two general practices in the south of England were invited, by letter, to use a testing kit. Only about 40% agreed to do so. The rest were interviewed to find out why they had not accepted the invitation: reasons given included distaste or embarrassment about the procedure, lack of time, and variants of 'I don't want to know' or 'it can't happen to me'.

## PSYCHOLOGICAL DRAWBACKS OF SCREENING

Screening advice occasionally precipitates unnecessary obsessional worries about cancer in a healthy person. For certain sections of the population in which the risk of finding cancer is small, screening programmes may do more harm than good.

Breast screening for women under 35, for example (Frank and Mai, 1985), often results in the discovery of small breast lumps. Though the vast majority of lumps in this age group are benign, it is necessary to carry out hospital investigations to make quite sure that the occasional malignant lump is not missed. Such investigations cause many women extreme anxiety, quite apart from the time and expense they entail.

# 7. Delay in Reporting Cancer Symptoms

Fear of cancer, and ignorance about its symptoms, can both lead patients to delay seeking medical attention. Fear of cancer is sometimes conscious: 'I couldn't tell my doctor because I was terrified I'd got cancer.' Sometimes it is unconscious, and the patient uses the mental mechanism of 'denial' as protection against overwhelming anxiety. Denial, which is a psychoanalytic term meaning failure to take in some threatening aspect of reality, cannot be directly observed, and this term is therefore used much more freely by some people than others. Denial about cancer may be inferred if a patient seems unaware of obvious evidence of serious disease, or inappropriately unconcerned about it. For example, a woman who is found to have a large or ulcerating breast tumour during a medical examination carried out for some other reason, and who claims she has never noticed anything wrong with her breast before, could be using denial. Alternatively, she could have deliberately concealed her tumour but did not like to admit it. (Denial in this context has harmful results but denial in other circumstances may work to patients' benefit, as discussed in later sections.)

Ignorance about the symptoms of cancer is still widespread. Lumps and bleeding are recognized as potentially serious by most people, but other presentations of the disease may not be. Virtually all women know that a lump in the breast may mean cancer, but many women do not attach so much importance to another breast symptom such as a change in shape.

Delay and the reasons for it were studied in a series of 314 patients with various types of cancer presenting to a hospital in Manchester (Aitken-Swan and Paterson, 1955). Nearly half had delayed at least three months between noticing their first symptom and seeking medical advice. Sometimes the delay had been due to ignorance, that is, failure to realize that an initially trivial symptom might signify serious disease. The longest delays, however, were due to fear, in patients who did suspect they had cancer.

One might have expected that both ignorance and fear would have diminished considerably in the 30 years since this work was done, for information about cancer is far more freely available now, but more recent studies show that delay in presentation remains common. A survey of new patients referred to the breast clinic in Southampton (Nichols *et al.*, 1981) found that older women delayed longer than younger ones, and women with breast cancer delayed longer than those with benign breast disease. The latter finding suggests that women with breast lumps often have correct suspicions about whether they have cancer or not before they consult a doctor. The survey was followed by a public health education campaign about breast disease, directed at both the general public and at general practitioners (Waters *et al.*, 1983), but delay in referral to the breast clinic is still common.

Combining two breast cancer research series of my own, 41 patients — nearly half the total of 84 — admitted to a delay of at least six weeks. For nine of them, delay had been over a year. The chief reasons for delay were classified as follows:

*The first symptom was not a lump:* 12 patients. 'The nipple did seem a different shape, but I thought it was nothing to worry about. If there'd been a lump there I'd have thought about cancer and gone to my doctor straight away.' Such cases may reflect a true deficit in public health education, for these patients said they thought the first symptom of breast cancer was always a lump. This statement may, however, have been used as an excuse.

*Conscious fear or worry:* 10 patients. Fear of having cancer was more often mentioned than fear of having a mastectomy.

*General practitioner delay:* 8 patients. These women had been advised not to worry when they first went to their GPs, and had usually hesitated to return for several months although the breast abnormality was becoming more obvious.

*Probable denial:* 7 patients.

'I wasn't sure if it was anything.'
'I didn't take much notice.'
'I just put it off.'
'You don't take any notice.'
'I thought everyone had lumps like this.'
'I don't believe in searching for nasties.'
'My doctor said it must have been there a long time but I never noticed it.'

Many of these statements are rather vague and illustrate the difficulty of distinguishing denial from ignorance or from deliberate suppression of concern.

*No reason given:* 4 patients.

The role of 'ego defence mechanisms' in causing delay is discussed in a study of 90 women admitted to an Australian hospital for biopsy of a breast lump (Magarey *et al.,* 1977). From video recordings of long unstructured interviews with these patients, these authors concluded that use of psychological processes like denial and suppression made a greater contribution to delay than more readily measurable factors like age, education, and knowledge about cancer, and that denial and suppression were also more important in this respect than fear of cancer or mastectomy. How denial and suppression were assessed, however, is not stated in practical reproducible terms. The women who had delayed seeking medical advice in this series obtained lower anxiety scores on a questionnaire than those who had presented promptly, but they were said to appear more anxious at interview. They were more depressed than the rest on various measures. In discussion, the authors suggest that the type of patient who deals with the threat of disease by denial, suppression and avoidance will ignore straightforward health education programmes in the same way. The remedy is not obvious, but they suggest more subtle health education measures using thesort of techniques developed in advertising, also that doctors ought to take the initiative in carrying out 'routine' examinations of patients' breasts rather than leaving it to the patients to report abnormalities.

Many studies on delay have focused on breast cancer, because delay is easy to measure in this condition: the patient can often pinpoint a specific occasion when she noticed the lump or other change in the breast. For other types of cancer, 'delay' and 'denial' are harder to assess, because the symptoms develop gradually and are not dramatic at first; symptoms like tiredness, weakness, weight loss or poor appetite, 'indigestion' or change of bowel habit, cough or shortness of breath, especially in older people, may go on getting worse for several months before either patient or doctor suspects anything seriously wrong, and it is impossible to date their onset accurately.

Delay in diagnosis of cancer can be the responsibility of the doctor rather than the patient. Sometimes, as when the doctor has not done a proper examination or is unaware of the significance of the patient's symptoms and signs, there is no excuse. In other cases the doctor fails to make the right diagnosis at first because the symptoms and signs are indistinguishable from a much commoner benign (non-cancerous) condition. Unconscious mental mechanisms can be used by doctors as well as patients, and one could postulate that 'denial' leads some doctors to ignore evidence suggesting cancer in patients they like, or with whom they identify as being in some way similar to themselves.

## PROMPT PRESENTATION

Anxiety has been considered above as one of the causes of delay, but anxiety may equally well have the reverse effect of spurring patients to seek immediate medical attention if they develop symptoms which they suspect are due to cancer. Patients who respond in this way often demand immediate treatment, and understandably find it very difficult to tolerate the delays of a few days or weeks which usually elapse in the National Health Service before hospital investigations for urgent but non-emergency cases can be arranged.

## SUMMARY

Patients often delay for weeks or months, and occasionally for years, in reporting signs or symptoms of cancer, and their chances of cure are reduced as a result. The main reasons for delay are ignorance and anxiety; some writers also attribute great importance to the unconscious mental mechanism of 'denial'. How far public health education can eliminate delay remains uncertain.

# 8. False Alarms, Hypochondriasis and Cancer Phobia

Excessive fear of cancer among people who do not have this disease justifies brief consideration here. Some people who consult their doctors because they are afraid they have developed cancer are really suffering from psychological disorders, which have caused very minor physical symptoms to take on a sinister significance in their minds. The psychological background to such cases is often never recognized, but even if it is, hospital investigations are often arranged 'just to be on the safe side'.

About a third of those patients in my research studies who had been referred to hospital with suspected lung or breast cancer, but in whom no evidence of cancer was found, reported psychological problems during the previous year: a high proportion. The cancer scare often followed on from the psychological problem:

1. *A single man in his late 40's, always anxious and obsessional by nature, felt plagued by indecision as to whether or not he wanted to marry his girlfriend. He became increasingly introspective and depressed. When he told his doctor he was coughing up blood and thought he had lung cancer, he was admitted to hospital, but then admitted he had merely panicked about slight bleeding from his gums after brushing his teeth too hard. Nothing physically wrong was found.*
2. *A married woman in her 50's had been severely depressed for two years for no apparent reason, and made no improvement after trials of various antidepressant drugs. She noticed a small lump in her breast and asked to have it examined by a specialist, since she had heard about several cases of breast*

*cancer among her acquaintances. During the research interview she said she did not really think the lump was anything unusual, and attendance at the breast clinic confirmed that the mild nodularity of her breasts was within normal limits. This patient had a long history of recurrent depression, had attended a great many hospital departments in the past, and had many surgical operations.*

In the following case, though the patient himself was not worried about cancer, his doctors were understandably misled by the similarity between the symptoms of cancer and the symptoms of depression:

*A man in his 60's attended the chest clinic regularly because he had chronic bronchitis. On one of his routine visits he said his usual cough and shortness of breath were more troublesome, and he also complained of losing weight and having headaches. He was admitted to the chest hospital for investigation, for a diagnosis of lung cancer with cerebral metastases seemed quite likely. No cancer was detected, however, and observation on the ward made it clear he was severely depressed: the weight loss and headaches were symptoms of a depressive illness. He was treated with the antidepressant drug amitriptyline and made a good recovery.*

Depressive illnesses and anxiety states are the commonest formal psychiatric diagnoses in cases of this kind. Occasionally, delusions (false beliefs) or hallucinations (false perceptions) on the theme of having cancer arise in patients with a severe mental illness such as schizophrenia. However, many of those patients who develop groundless fears of cancer are not mentally ill in the formal sense: they are anxious, unhappy people, perhaps recently upset by having had a relative or friend suffer from cancer, or just going through a 'bad patch' in their own lives for some other reason. Some patients of this kind are genuinely convinced they have cancer. Others are quite thankful to admit their problems are psychological if this possibility is put to them sympathetically, although they have found it easier to present a physical symptom to their doctors than reveal psychological worries straight away.

This section has been designed to draw attention to an important minority of patients. They easily go unrecognized in busy clinics, because doctors do not realize the psychological background to their complaints. Therefore some of them repeatedly undergo time-consuming and expensive X-rays or surgical procedures with negative results, and never receive appropriate treatment for their mental problems. I do not wish to imply that everyone who is investigated for cancer but proved not to have it is mentally ill or a hypochondriac: many such patients have perfectly genuine physical symptoms or signs which merit investigation, and some turn out to have another physical disease which needs treatment.

# 9. Reactions to a Suspected Diagnosis of Cancer

Different patients' responses to a suspected diagnosis of cancer range from resigned acceptance to mental agony. The nature of an individual patient's reaction is influenced by personality and current circumstances, and of course it depends on how well informed the patient is about the illness.

## REACTION PATTERNS

The following classification, which could be applied to any other serious physical disease besides cancer, is based on the description by Lloyd (1977).

*Calm acceptance.* 'I know it could be cancer, but I don't mind if it is.' 'You can't change what's meant to be. After all, I've had a good life.' About half the patients in my studies of both lung cancer and breast cancer seemed calm, resigned and unconcerned at the time of their first referral to hospital, even though they appreciated they probably had a serious illness. This reaction is most frequent in those who have stable, stoic personalities, who consider they have already lived a fulfilling life and are now ready to draw it to a close, and in those with strong religious faith.

*Denial.* 'He said I'd better just come in for a checkup, but I know it isn't anything much.' Though patients like this, by agreeing to come into hospital, have acknowledged some possibility of something wrong, they do not admit it could be serious. Such patients do not ask questions of their doctors, and they fail to 'take in' any hints, or even direct information that they are given about the true state of affairs. Denial probably comes most naturally to patients who are elderly or have little education, but it is sometimes found in intelligent articulate people who need to defend themselves against intolerable anxiety or despair.

*Anxiety.* This may be focused on one specific aspect of the illness:

'I've always had a dread of cancer.'

'I don't mind about having cancer, I'm just terrified they'll say I need the breast off.'

'It's all right with me if they do take the breast off. What scares me is the thought of that radium treatment.'

'It doesn't matter about me, but I'm worried sick about the wife — what's going to happen if I'm not there to look after her?'

*Depression.* Depression and anxiety are often mixed. If mild cases are included, about one-third of my research patients were depressed when they presented to hospital. In the lung cancer series, depression was more common in patients whose tumour was far advanced or whose physical state was poor, but seldom seemed to be solely the result of the physical illness; most of the severely depressed patients had current social problems and/or a past history of depression as well.

*A retired businessman aged 70, widowed nine years earlier, had five months' history of pain in the shoulders and shortness of breath. His GP's referral letter described him as an obsessional person who had often attended surgery over the years with symptoms of depression or anxiety. During the research interview he described many depressive symptoms which he said had started two years previously, after the death of his beloved dog had left him living alone. His depression had got worse as his physical symptoms developed. He was found to have an anaplastic carcinoma of the lung, complicated by carcinomatous neuromyopathy.*

*Guilt and Stigma.* 'I know this must be a punishment for something. I suppose I haven't lived such a good life as I should.'

'I feel like a leper — I dread anyone finding out I've got cancer, I'm so ashamed.'

Patients who show such reactions are often depressed. For some patients, the absence of a convincing medical explanation as to why they should have been 'singled out' to develop cancer leads them to lay the blame on their own bad behaviour in the past.

*Anger.* Patients' distress may be projected onto other people, for example they blame the doctor who failed to make the correct diagnosis right at the start, or the employer who was responsible for exposing them to toxic chemicals: patients who respond this way refuse to accept that a factor like their own heavy smoking can have played any part in their illness.

These reaction patterns are not fixed, for any one patient may display a mixture at one time, or pass through several stages. A patient may, for example, respond to the first symptoms of cancer with denial, then go through a period of depression or anxiety when the symptoms become too marked to ignore, but finally achieve an attitude of realistic acceptance. Distressed patients often become calmer once they know the facts about their illness, for most patients find unconfirmed suspicions of the worst are harder to bear than certainty even if the truth is unpleasant. Waiting a few days for the result of a biopsy or X-ray can seem an endless ordeal, and staff do not always realize that patients find such delays distressing even if knowing the result more quickly would make no difference to the treatment plan or eventual prognosis.

## DOCTOR-PATIENT COMMUNICATION ABOUT THE SUSPECTED DIAGNOSIS

Reactions to a suspected diagnosis of cancer depend, of course, whether the patient is aware of the likelihood of cancer at all, and if so, how far he or she appreciates what this means in terms of treatment and prognosis. These things in turn depend on the patient's knowledge about cancer in general, and how much discussion with doctors about his or her individual case has taken place.

I asked 138 lung cancer patients, about to have a bronchoscopy to confirm the diagnosis, 'What have the doctors said is likely to be wrong?' About one-third of the group spontaneously mentioned 'cancer', and of these, about half seemed quite philosophical about the matter:

'I think it's cancer, but I don't mind if it is.'
'I've a feeling it could be a touch of cancer. I'm tough — I can accept death. Now I'm 70, when my number's up it's up.'
'It's funny, I always said I'd shoot myself if I got cancer, but now it doesn't worry me at all.'

Some patients of this kind had discussed cancer with their doctors, others had not apparently wanted to do so, as they had accepted the possibility with fatalism or even indifference, or did not consider it their place to ask for information: 'The doctor's the kingpin — he knows what's right to tell you, more often than not.'

The other half of the group who mentioned 'cancer' were anxious or depressed at the prospect. Few of them had managed to discuss their concerns in an open fashion. Some were ambivalent about whether they wanted information, or felt they had not been given straight answers to their questions:

'I think I've got cancer, but the doctors haven't said so and I don't want to know. I'm terrified — petrified — of that damn sickness.'
'They say they don't know, but it's obvious they're pulling the wool over my eyes — it's got to be cancer.'
'I asked him frankly if it was TB or cancer and he said "Well, it's not TB".'
'After the usual lot of hooey I deduced it was cancer. He admitted they couldn't rule it out.'
'At first I was afraid it was cancer, but now he's put my mind at rest.'

Some of the patients who did not mention cancer in response to my question may have had suspicions about it which they did not want to discuss, or even admit to themselves. Some gave strong hints that they might have a serious illness:

'I don't think I'm going to get better.'
'If it's there it's there.'
'The doctors are here to put you right, but if they can't it's just too bad.'
'When my time comes I shall go.'
Others just repeated a medical term like 'a shadow on the lung', 'congestion', 'a cyst'. 'inflammation', even 'he said it was a blank.' They showed no curiosity about what these terms really meant.
A small proportion of patients, whether because of ignorance or complete denial, said they had no idea at all but they were sure it was nothing serious:
'I'm perfect for my age.'
'I've got powerful intuition, and I know I'm all right.'

Superficially, these findings suggest a large deficit in doctor-patient communication, but this interpretation is too simple. Doctors may be rightly reluctant to raise the question of cancer before the diagnosis is certain, for some patients who have a bronchoscopy for suspected lung cancer turn out to have other, less serious, chest conditions. Some of the patients who complained about doctors' evasiveness might have forgotten or misinterpreted what they had been told, because they were ambivalent about wanting to hear it, or projected their own reluctance to discuss diagnosis onto the doctors. Doctor-patient communication later in the course of the illness, after the diagnosis is confirmed and while treatment is being given, will be considered in Section II.6.

Finally, I will summarize a study carried out on 50 newly diagnosed cancer patients who were about to begin radiotherapy in a New York hospital (Peck, 1972). Forty knew they had cancer but only 14 had been told this by a doctor and the other 26 had guessed their diagnosis from the various medical procedures which had been done. In response to the illness, various emotions were displayed: anxiety (41 patients), depression (18 patients), guilt (18 patients), anger (22 patients). The emotional reaction was only judged severe enough to merit psychiatric intervention in one case. Four patients spoke of suicide, but none made or planned a suicide attempt. The mental defence mechanisms shown by these patients included denial, relating more to the prognosis than to the diagnosis itself; equating cancer to other diseases they had recovered from in the past; learning all about cancer so they could play an active part in their own treatment and that of others; and attributing wonderful powers to modern medicine.

# PART II: LIVING WITH CANCER AND ITS TREATMENT

# 1. Introduction

This middle part of the book deals with the first few months after the diagnosis of cancer has been made. During this period, most patients will have to make psychological adjustments. Treatment may be demanding and give rise to side-effects. There will be uncertainty about the future outcome of the illness. Roles at home and work, and relationships with family and friends, are changed.

Three main kinds of treatment, surgery, radiotherapy, and chemotherapy (drug treatment), are used alone or in combination for the treatment of cancer. Curative, or radical, treatment is designed to achieve complete elimination of the cancer: many curative regimes have to be quite drastic if they are to succeed in this aim, and often have marked side-effects. Palliative treatment, in contrast, is a gentler affair, designed to relieve symptoms or prolong life for a while when the cancer is too advanced to be cured. Whether a treatment is curative or palliative, its benefits must be measured against its side-effects in deciding whether it is worthwhile. The psychological consequences of various regimes should carry much weight in these decisions.

A significant minority of patients suffering from cancer become clinically depressed and in the section on depression I will describe the diagnosis, frequency, and management of this common psychiatric disorder as it occurs in the cancer treatment setting. Other patients, the majority, escape depression and make a good psychological adaptation to their illness: I will examine the mental strategies which enable them to do so.

Cancer patients' relaitionship with other people may be a

source of problems as well as support. The question of doctor-patient communication, and how far patients wish to be informed about their illness, is relevant here. Relatives, besides providing support for the patients, often have emotional problems of their own.

The last section in this part of the book examines some evidence on whether psychological counselling can help to prevent the emotional distress which cancer patients might otherwise endure.

# 2. Surgery

For some types of cancer, any surgical operation which is to succeed in achieving a cure has to be extensive, removing a large margin of healthy tissue surrounding the tumour, even removing the whole of the organ in which the tumour lies. Other types of cancer can be cured by smaller operations, often followed by radiotherapy or cytotoxic drugs.

Major cancer surgery can leave the patient with an obvious defect in physical appearance or function or both: for example, removal of the breast (mastectomy), stomach (gastrectomy), large bowel (colectomy), womb and ovaries (hysterectomy and oophorectomy), or amputation of a limb. Such defects are inevitably distressing, but most patients are prepared to accept an operation which causes considerable mutilation or disablement, if the alternative is to die from cancer. People who oppose these drastic operations may not realize that untreated, or inadequately treated, cancers give rise to even more horrible defects of appearance or function, for example an infected ulcerating growth destroying a visible part of the body, or paraplegia from a secondary deposit beside the spinal cord.

While the physical defects produced by major surgery may be justifiably regarded as a necessary evil, the price which sometimes has to be paid for cure, it is not justifiable to ignore or dismiss the psychological distress which many patients suffer as a result of these defects. Research shows that such distress can be lessened by appropriate management, as discussed at the end of this section.

Mastectomy for breast cancer has received much more attention from the psychological viewpoint than any other kind of cancer surgery, because it poses an obvious threat to 'body image' and sexual attractiveness. Other cancer operations, less extensively studied, cause greater defects of appearance and function and might have even greater potential for causing psychological distress.

## MASTECTOMY

In the year after mastectomy, a quarter to a third of women will experience significant depression, anxiety or sexual dysfunction (Morris *et al.,* 1977; Maguire *et al.,* 1978). Sometimes, however, these problems are due to concern about future recurrence of cancer rather than to the operation itself. Distress following mastectomy has received a great deal of emphasis in recent years, both in the medical press and in the 'media', to the point where the case against this operation has probably been exaggerated. Of 44 women I followed up for 9-12 months after mastectomy for breast cancer in 1980, only six described severe and lasting distress about this particular aspect of their illness or its treatment. Two examples follow.

1. *(Divorced, early 60's) She expressed profound sadness at the preoperative interview about the prospect of losing a breast. For several months postoperatively, she described feeling 'a freak' and said the operation 'had accentuated getting old'. She found the scar and the prosthesis distasteful and avoided looking at them. She also avoided the sports and social activities she had previously enjoyed, because they required revealing clothing. She apologized for her reaction: 'I really shouldn't mind at my age, especially when I haven't got a husband.' There was some improvement by the time of the final follow-up.*

2. *(Married, late 40's) 'Terrified' about mastectomy at the preoperative interview. After the operation she delayed six weeks before she could bring herself to look at the scar and, because she felt so disfigured, she never let her husband see it at all. She did not leave the house for weeks, and could not go back to work for six months. By the end of the year she*

*felt better, and described the whole experience as a tremendous mental and physical trauma from which she had emerged a stronger person.*

Women who are badly upset by mastectomy may be married or single, old or young, but in this and other studies can usually be picked out in advance by their marked aversion to the prospect of the operation.

The other 38 women in my study managed to adapt to their mastectomy quite quickly, though many of them were distressed for the first few weeks, as illustrated by the following case.

*(Married, late 40's) She had some tearful spells in the first fortnight but felt sustained by her determination to get better and by her family's encouragement. Over the next few months she experienced occasional distress, for example when finding a low-cut dress she could no longer wear, but six months after the operation was confident she had 'fully accepted' the mastectomy. Her husband's support made her feel 'a complete woman' and she was delighted with her prosthesis. When offered breast reconstruction by plastic surgery, she decided it was not worth the bother.*

Sexual problems following mastectomy usually affect women who already lack confidence or who already have some difficulties in this area. Half the 30 married women in my series made a point of showing their husbands their mastectomy scar at an early stage, and all of them felt he had accepted the experience well. The others were embarrassed to reveal their disfigurement: in some cases this was not of great importance because the couple were elderly and no longer sexually active, but for some of the others it led to marital difficulties. Two of the younger women in the series, one widowed and one divorced, were hoping to find a new sexual partner. Neither was particularly upset by the mastectomy on her own account, but both feared it would prove a barrier to any new sexual relationship. Both women did break up with a boyfriend during the follow-up period, and it is interesting to speculate how far this was due to their own expectations of failure, and how far to the man's true reaction. The younger of these two women, who was in her early thirties, overcame the problem and became engaged to another man six months after her operation.

Nearly half the whole group claimed they were hardly distressed by the mastectomy at all. These women volunteered various explanations for their ability to accept an operation which they knew many women would consider an appalling disfigurement.

'It's not a problem to lose a breast at my age.'
'Almost a relief not to have any more worries about lumpy breasts.'
'Life's more important than breasts.'
'I've got such a good husband it doesn't make any difference.'
'I haven't got a husband, so I needn't worry.'
'People can't see it.'
'Not so bad as losing a useful bit like an arm or leg.'

Some people would not take such responses at face value, but label them examples of 'denial' or 'rationalization' to mask the patients' true feelings of profound despair. There is no evidence that this speculation is correct: many patients adapt much better than certain psychologically-minded professionals like to believe!

## COLOSTOMY

The operation of colostomy involves removing the rectum and part of the large bowel, so excretion of faeces takes place through an artificial opening on the abdomen. To investigate the psychological and social aftermath of this operation, 83 patients in London and Southend who had had a colostomy for cancer 1-8 years earlier were interviewed (Devlin *et al.*, 1971). Depression was common, as were major practical problems like unemployment resulting from the operation, or lack of facilities to dispose of dressings. Half the sample had sexual difficulties, blamed partly on damage to the pelvic nerves during surgery and partly on distaste and embarrassment in patients or their partners. Many patients had little contact, or inadequate communication, with their GP or district nurse.

## LARYNGECTOMY

Laryngectomy — removal of the larynx or 'voicebox' — is sometimes required to cure cancer of the throat. The chief handicap resulting from this operation is loss of normal speech, though many patients can learn good 'oesophageal speech.' Follow-up of 50 consecutive patients who had a laryngectomy in a Californian clinic (Barton, 1965) suggests an adverse psychological outcome from this operation is common. Five patients had committed suicide, at times ranging from two months to eight years postoperatively. Four had died from alcoholism and eight were drinking very heavily. Only eight were considered 'well and adjusted.' This poor outcome can only partly be attributed to the operation itself, for heavy drinking and smoking contribute to development of laryngeal cancer, and might have been associated with a pre-existing psychological disturbance.

## LUNG SURGERY

Not all major cancer operations cause distress. The lung cancer patients in my research series who had the affected lung partly or entirely removed (lobectomy or pneumonectomy) all considered the operation well worth while and none had found it particularly gruelling. None were depressed. The belief that the operation had cured them seemed partly responsible for their good adjustment, though for most it was to prove unjustified.

## PREVENTING PSYCHOLOGICAL PROBLEMS AFTER CANCER SURGERY

Some patients will inevitably be distressed by mutilating or disabling surgery. Doctors can help to reduce such distress by giving clear explanations of the operation and its consequences beforehand, making sure that patients have access to any necessary practical aids and understand how to use them, and allowing patients clear opportunities to ask questions or raise problems at any stage. Patients who do develop problems may benefit from referral to a specialist such as a psychiatrist, psychologist or social worker, and the need for such referrals should not be seen as anything extraordinary or shameful.

Counselling by a specialized nurse is now offered as a routine part of the care of mastectomy patients in many centres in Britain, and some centres also employ nurse-counsellors with special knowledge of other cancer operations. Counselling may also be offered by a patient who has made a good adaptation to the same operation in the past. Counselling may be carried out individually or in small groups and involves giving practical information as well as offering psychological benefits, for example demonstrating that others have successfully overcome handicaps similar to those which the newly diagnosed patient might consider overwhelming. Not all patients want counselling, and a few are upset by it, but most find it beneficial. The psychological aspects of counselling are discussed in more detail in Section II.8.

The current trend to take patients' psychological responses into account when evaluating different treatments is a welcome one, so long as it is remembered that different patients react to the same operation in such varied ways that simple generalizations are not useful in every case. For breast cancer, for example, growing awareness that mastectomy often leads to anxiety, depression, and sexual problems helped to stimulate research into alternative methods of treatment, and there is now evidence that a smaller operation ('lumpectomy') followed by radiotherapy to the remaining breast tissue is just as effective as mastectomy in achieving cure for some early cancers of the breast. An alternative means of preserving the appearance of the breast is to reconstruct this organ by plastic surgery, either at the same time as mastectomy or a few months later. Studies of women who have a lumpectomy (Steinburg *et al.,* 1985) or breast reconstruction (Dean *et al.,* 1983) suggest that they are less likely to develop psychological problems than those treated by mastectomy alone. But individual patients can prove exceptions. If given a choice about their treatment some patients choose mastectomy, because they would feel more confident of recovery if they were completely rid of a diseased body part, or because they do not want to have radiotherapy after the operation. Another example is provided by a finding from an American clinical trial on the treatment of limb sarcomas (Sugarbaker *et al.,* 1981), in which amputation followed by chemotherapy was compared with more limited surgery followed by both chemotherapy and radiotherapy. Patients who had the limb amputated were rather better psychologically adjusted afterwards: the others complained their preserved limb was painful and useless.

There will always be a few patients for whom a particular surgical operation is a psychological disaster, however much effort is devoted to helping them cope. Patients like this can often be identified in advance by their extreme fear at the prospect of the operation, and some of them will be better off with another type of treatment even if it does not give them such a good physical prognosis. Most patients with cancer, however, are willing and able to accept the adverse effects of major surgery if it offers them the best available hope of cure.

# 3. Radiotherapy

Radiotherapy is the use of high energy irradiation to destroy unwanted tissue, and its main use is in the treatment of cancer. Like other forms of cancer treatment, radiotherapy may be 'radical' or 'palliative'. Radical radiotherapy, given with the aim of cure, is the most suitable treatment for certain types of cancer which are highly sensitive to radiation, or for tumours which would be difficult or impossible to remove by surgery because they occupy an awkward position in the body. Palliative radiotherapy, given when the cancer is too advanced for cure, often brings worthwhile benefits like controlling pain, or shrinking a tumour mass which was hampering a vital function like breathing or swallowing. Another term is 'adjuvant' radiotherapy, treatment given as a preventive measure after a limited surgical operation such as 'lumpectomy' for breast cancer, which has probably left some of the tumour behind.

Most radiotherapy is delivered by an 'external beam', which is applied in a variable number of 'fractions', several times a week over several weeks, because giving the whole dose at once would cause too much damage to healthy parts of the body. Less commonly, radiotherapy is delivered by an 'implant', that is a small source of radioactive metal is left inside the tumour itself for a few hours or days.

Side-effects of radiotherapy arise because the treatment causes cell destruction, affecting normal cells as well as cancer cells. Tiredness, nausea, and burning of the skin are common short-term side-effects, and many others may develop depending on what part of the body is being treated: for example treatment to the abdomen causes diarrhoea, and treatment to the head causes hair loss. These effects are generally worst towards the end of treatment and for a few weeks afterwards, and they recover within the following few weeks. Long-term side-effects, developing months or years later, are generally due to fibrosis of tissue in the treated areas.

## PSYCHOLOGICAL STUDIES OF PATIENTS RECEIVING RADIOTHERAPY

Radical, palliative, and adjuvant radiotherapy differ in their psychological impact. Patients receiving radical treatment in the expectation of cure can often cheerfully accept long courses with marked side-effects of a kind which patients on palliative treatment would find hard to tolerate. Adjuvant radiotherapy may seem especially demanding because it has no obvious short-term physical benefits to compensate for its side-effects and inconvenience.

Many people dread the prospect of radiotherapy because they associate it with incurable cancer, or regard radioactivity as a dangerous mystery. Fifty patients receiving radiotherapy for various types of cancer in New York were interviewed before and after treatment (Peck and Boland, 1977). Beforehand, most of them displayed much ignorance about radiotherapy, and the beliefs they did possess were unduly pessimistic, for example they did not realize that some forms of cancer can be cured by this treatment. A week after their course finished, only one-third of these patients felt any better; two-thirds were physically worse because of radiation side-effects, and the frequency of depression and anxiety among them had increased. An interview at a later stage would undoubtedly have revealed a happier result, for 60% of these patients were free of any sign of recurrent cancer two or three years later.

The psychological effects of the actual process of receiving external beam radiotherapy, which involves being left alone in a room with a large machine in an immobile posture, were investigated by comparing two groups, each consisting of 100 patients, treated by two different machines (Forester *et al.*, 1978). Patients treated with the betatron, a large and noisy machine on which every session could take up to half an hour, reported more mood disturbance during their course than those treated with the linear accelerator, a smaller and quieter machine on which each session took only a few minutes. By the end of the course, however, mood disturbance was equally frequent in both groups.

Twenty-four of my research patients with incurable lung cancer had palliative radiotherapy to the chest, and were interviewed about a month after the course finished. Their opinions of radiotherapy were favourable. Seventeen considered it 'definitely worthwhile', four 'probably worthwhile', and three were uncertain, but nobody regretted having it. Some patients praised radiotherapy because it had improved or abolished physical symptoms like cough, breathlessness or chest pain. Other patients, even though their physical state was not improved, still spoke well of radiotherapy, because they were pleased to have 'had something done' or because they appreciated the radiographers' kindness.

Experience of side-effects varied a great deal although all the patients had been given similar treatment regimes. About half said they had no side-effects to speak of. One man said 'Nothing to it, I enjoyed it. I wish I could have some more.' Among the rest, the commonest 'worst side-effect' was a mixture of physical weakness and mental malaise, often including depressed mood or tearfulness, lasting a few hours after each treatment. Sustained depression arising for the first time during the course of radiotherapy was not found among this sample of patients. Those who were already depressed beforehand said they felt even worse as a result of the debilitating effects of treatment, yet their mood usually improved when the course was over and they noticed its physical benefits, as illustrated by the following case.

*A married man in his late 40's had been depressed for a year before his lung cancer was diagnosed, and put this down to the 'anguish' of being unemployed for the first time in his life. His tumour was too advanced to be curable by surgery, and he was given a course of palliative radiotherapy to relieve the severe pain in his chest. He said of this treatment: 'I found it very, very hard to cope with, but I got through because they'd warned me what to expect. All the energy drained out of me afterwards, and then the tears broke.' By the end of the course his pain had improved 'like a miracle' and his depressive symptoms were not so bad as they had been when he first presented.*

## LATE SIDE-EFFECTS

For patients who survive years after having radiotherapy, there may be permanent physical effects on the part of the body which was treated, and these sometimes have psychological consequences.

Radiation fibrosis is a common cause of late side-effects. For example, radiotherapy for cancer of the cervix can cause shortening, narrowing, and dryness of the vagina, and therefore impair sexual function. Patients with this difficulty in one study (Seibel *et al.,* 1980) had seldom mentioned it during their 'routine' follow-up care, though they might have been helped by advice on the use of lubricants, and reassurance that intercourse would not cause further physical damage.

Increasing numbers of children and young adults now survive into adult life after having radical radiotherapy as part of their treatment for leukaemia, lymphoma, or some solid tumours. Radiotherapy to the developing brain causes subtle behavioural and intellectual changes (Chessells, 1985). Radiotherapy to the reproductive organs may cause infertility and consequent psychological distress.

Problems like these, though nearly everyone would think them worth putting up with for the sake of curing the cancer and in consequence some patients feel they will appear ungrateful if they complain, deserve attention. If problems have already developed, there are sometimes ways of lessening them. Better still, it may be possible to devise improvements in technique which will prevent similar problems altogether for patients being treated in the future.

# 4. Chemotherapy

Chemotherapy means drug treatment. In cancer work, 'chemotherapy' is usually used as a shorthand for cytotoxic drug treatment, with which most of this section is concerned. Hormone treatment will be briefly mentioned at the end.

Cytotoxic drugs kill body cells, including both cancer cells and normal cells. Several types exist, each acting in a different way, and the most effective method of using cytotoxic drugs is to give a mixture of several types at once: 'combination chemotherapy'. Most drugs of this kind have to be given by injection into a vein (intravenously), and treatment is usually divided into a number of 'pulses' or 'cycles', given a few weeks apart, so the normal cells have a chance to recover in between.

Side-effects of cytotoxic chemotherapy vary slightly depending on which drugs are being used, but common ones are tiredness, nausea and vomiting, diarrhoea, sore mouth, loss of hair, and lowering of the blood count which reduces resistance to infection.

Depression and anxiety among patients receiving chemotherapy is usually best explained as a reaction to the unpleasant physical side-effects of the treatment. Some patients feel so anxious about the nausea and vomiting associated with the injections that they are sick when injections are due, before any drug has actually been given. Some cytotoxic drugs have direct actions on the brain which alter mood, or disturb intellectual function causing cognitive impairment (Silberfarb *et al.,* 1980).

Chemotherapy regimes, like radiotherapy ones, include three broad categories depending upon the aim of treatment: curative, palliative, or adjuvant and each will be considered in turn.

## CURATIVE REGIMES

Advances in chemotherapy technique during recent years have been impressive. Certain cancers, including childhood leukaemia, lymphomas like Hodgkin's disease, and testicular tumours, can often be cured by chemotherapy alone. Curative regimes usually need to employ high doses of drugs, up to the limit which the normal cells of the body can tolerate, causing severe side-effects. Such regimes are therefore bound to be a considerable ordeal, but most patients are willingly prepared to tolerate this if treatment offers them a good chance of cure.

A study of 61 lymphoma patients in Wisconsin (Nerenz *et al.*, 1982) found emotional distress during chemotherapy was most severe for those patients whose disease responded rapidly to the treatment. This rather surprising finding could be explained physiologically, the result of the body's having to cope with a large load of tumour breakdown products, or it could have been due to the need for unexpectedly sudden psychological adjustment. Emotional distress was also more common among patients who reported a large number of physical side-effects, especially 'vague long-term' effects like tiredness and weakness which may be partly psychological in origin themselves.

## ADJUVANT CHEMOTHERAPY

Adjuvant chemotherapy, which entails giving cytotoxic drug treatment after a primary tumour has been surgically removed, has special psychological consequences. 'Adjuvant' patients have already had a major operation and no longer have any obvious evidence of cancer. They are advised to regard the chemotherapy as an 'insurance policy', which will diminish their chances of developing recurrent cancer in the future, but does not guarantee a cure. Many patients therefore consider adjuvant chemotherapy a burden, since it produces unpleasant side-effects without the compensation of any immediate tangible benefit, and also serves as an unwelcome reminder that the cancer might come back.

'Adjuvant' chemotherapy has been extensively used for breast cancer, especially for those patients who are known to have a substantial risk of recurrence after mastectomy because their axillary lymph nodes contain tumour deposits. Fifty patients having the 'CMF' regime (cyclophosphamide, methotrexate, and 5-fluorouracil) for this purpose in Los Angeles were interviewed (Meyerowitz *et al.*, 1979). All had unpleasant physical side-effects, and common psychological and social difficulties included nervousness, irritability, tearfulness, practical or financial problems, and adverse effects on relationships with family and friends. Although they all had difficulties, three-quarters of these women said they would recommend the same treatment to a friend in the same situation.

The psychological effect of the CMF regime was also studied in Manchester (Maguire *et al.*, 1980). Of 26 breast cancer patients receiving this treatment, 20 developed an anxiety state and 20 a depressive illness (some had both); a much greater psychiatric morbidity than that in the comparison patients treated by mastectomy alone. Anxiety and depression were most common among patients who had severe physical side-effects from their chemotherapy, and many of them had not disclosed the severity of these physical side-effects to the doctors looking after them.

Ten of the breast cancer patients I followed up after mastectomy were prescribed a six-month course of adjuvant chemotherapy. Without exception, these patients found chemotherapy very unpleasant, and all developed physical side-effects like vomiting, diarrhoea, and hair loss. Four were so distressed they did not complete the course. Four described severe depression lasting several days after each course, and one of these patients contemplated suicide. Two patients expressed puzzlement and distress about being given chemotherapy when they knew other patients did not have it. Two expressed loathing of the frequent visits to hospital, which retained unhappy associations for them however kindly they were treated in the chemotherapy clinic. Three spontaneously stated that the chemotherapy was much worse than the mastectomy and if this question had been routinely put to everybody, I think several others would have said the same.

## PALLIATIVE CHEMOTHERAPY

Twenty-one lung cancer patients in my research study were interviewed during the course of a chemotherapy regime, which usually consisted of cyclophosphamide, adriamycin, and VP16 given at three-weekly intervals. These patients had tumours of the 'oat-cell' histological type, which usually respond well to chemotherapy. Nine patients thought chemotherapy 'definitely worthwhile', another nine 'probably worthwhile', and three were uncertain, but none regretted having it. Even the few patients whose physical symptoms had failed to improve still considered chemotherapy worthwhile, because they hoped and believed it would do them good in the end: 'It's very rough, but I can take it — I'm determined to carry on.'

All these 21 patients found the side-effects of chemotherapy distressing. Nausea and vomiting was most often considered the worst side-effect, followed in frequency by general weakness. Hair loss, which doctors and nurses often regard as one of the worst side-effects of chemotherapy, affected all the patients, but most of the men said they did not mind it and only one woman regarded it as a really distressing effect.

Many patients described anxiety for several days before treatment, and depression for several days afterwards. For two patients, both of whom lived alone, this recurrent anxiety and depression were so bad they had to be admitted to hospital for every pulse of treatment. Five patients on chemotherapy had a sustained depressive illness, but there usually seemed to be other reasons for this besides the chemotherapy as shown by the following two cases.

1. *A widow of 60, who had had two previous episodes of depression in her life, had been depressed for some months when she first consulted her doctor about back pain, breathlessness, and cough. She thought her depression was due to loneliness and bad housing, made worse by her physical ill-health. Oat cell lung cancer was diagnosed, and chemotherapy prescribed. She developed intense anxiety lasting a week before each treatment, and for a week after each treatment her depression was more pronounced. The side-effects of nausea, vomiting, and hair loss caused her much distress. Despite the side-effects, she still thought treatment was worthwhile, because she knew her chest X-ray showed the tumour had shrunk. She still thought loneliness was the main reason for her depression.*

2. *A married man in his 50's presented with breathlessness, hoarse voice, and weight loss, and was found to have oat cell lung cancer. He accepted the diagnosis in a realistic manner, but said his wife and children had all been extremely upset and he was worried about whether they would be able to cope. At follow-up, he had received several cycles of chemotherapy without any improvement and had become depressed. The chemotherapy had produced severe vomiting and he felt generally 'rock bottom'. His wife, he said, was still very upset, convinced he would not get better, and he did not talk about his illness at home for fear of upsetting her further. He was trying to be optimistic and considered chemotherapy 'definitely worthwhile' because it gave him some hope for the future.*

A happier result is illustrated by the following case.

*A married man in his 40's became depressed when he found he had lung cancer, his main concern being the fear that he would not live to see his son established in a career. His tumour made a good response to chemotherapy and at follow-up his depression had recovered. Side-effects were severe, but he accepted this: 'It's one week out of three written off but that's not too bad, considering what's wrong.' On balance he felt 'on top of the world', with renewed hope for the future.*

The studies quoted show that most cancer patients are willing to put up with very unpleasant chemotherapy regimes, even if their benefits are not obvious. Sometimes the end results, whether palliation or cure, are well worthwhile. In other cases, the gruelling side-effects of this form of treatment are not justified in terms of the results, but many patients and doctors still feel obliged to persevere, to demonstrate their determination to combat the illness.

## HORMONE TREATMENT

Steroid hormones and related drugs, for example prednisolone and dexamethasone, are useful in treating many types of cancer. They have a direct effect on mood, the nature of which varies from patient to patient. The commonest mood change is a mild lifting of spirits and improvement of general well-being, and to most patients this is highly acceptable (Twycross and Guppy, 1985). Less often steroids have the undesirable effect of causing deep depression, exaggerated elation, or some other psychiatric disturbance. The physical effects of steroids in high doses include changing patients' appearance to produce the 'Cushingoid' pattern of bloated face and wasted limbs, which is often distressing.

The male and female sex hormones, androgens and oestrogens, influence the growth of some cancers, and treatment for these may entail altering sex hormone balance. Breast cancer and prostatic cancer are the most common tumours of this type. Inducing masculine secondary sex characteristics like a growth of body hair and a deep voice in women, or inducing impotence and breast enlargement in men, clearly has undesirable psychological consequences. The advent of drugs like tamoxifen, which change sex hormone function without causing side-effects, fortunately means that it is no longer necessary to subject many patients to these disturbing changes.

# 5. Attitudes and Coping Styles

When considering psychological responses to having cancer, there is a temptation to emphasize the problem cases: patients who become clinically depressed, patients whose lives are permanently shattered by the disease. Awareness of these problems is very important, but should not be allowed to obscure the fact that most cancer patients adapt to their illness remarkably well through the strength of their own personal resources, without professional help.

This chapter is largely concerned with what might be termed 'internal' mental attitudes. How well patients adapt to having cancer obviously depends too on other factors which, though they themselves are partly determined by mental attitude, will be considered separately in later sections. These other factors include how much the patients have been told about their illness, how much support they derive from their relationships with other people and from their religious beliefs, and whether they are clinically depressed.

According to a number of studies, patients with stable personalities and marriages, and those who have coped well with crises earlier in life, generally adapt to cancer and its treatment rather better than patients who have 'neurotic' personalities or a past history of psychiatric disturbance. The following stoic patient lived right through her illness without distress:

*A woman in her 70's had lived a contented uneventful life and always managed to 'accept things', including the death of her husband ten years before. She was referred to the chest hospital when she became short of breath, and at the first research interview just before diagnosis she remarked 'No good to worry, what will be will be' and scored zero on the depression questionnaire. Investigations showed she had lung cancer, but she was not told the diagnosis, and never asked. At follow-up she was more breathless but did not complain, and said 'I expect it will get better in time.' She died at home a few days later.*

In contrast, the next case history illustrates how an already vulnerable patient may break down completely under the stress of illness.

*A divorced male nurse of 60 had been depressed for about three years, during which time he had taken several overdoses and required psychiatric day care. The depression was thought to result from social isolation since his divorce and retirement. He then developed breathlessness and chest pain and was found to have lung cancer, for which chemotherapy was prescribed. At follow-up his depression was worse and he had spent some time as a psychiatric inpatient. He attributed the worsening of his depression to the chemotherapy, which terrified him, and caused extreme nausea and vomiting. However he considered this treatment well worthwhile because it had improved his chest pain. Although one of his doctors had spent a long time explaining his diagnosis and treatment, and he must have had some medical knowledge himself, he claimed to have been told nothing, and said he had asked no questions: 'they might think I was being nosy — it's probably none of my business.'*

Less commonly, the very opposite is found, and the diagnosis of cancer acts as a challenge which breaks a long pattern of poor adjustment, as in these two cases.

*1. A clerk aged 60, recently divorced, presented with one year's history of tiredness and coughing. He knew his chest X-ray showed 'a growth — something like a cancer.' For many years, on and off, he had been drinking heavily and feeling depressed, and had once made an attempt to gas himself with car exhaust fumes. Lung cancer was diagnosed and treated by surgical removal of the affected lung. Two months later his depression was much improved, he had become reunited with his wife, and had given up both drinking and smoking.*

*2. A 66-year-old married storeman had suffered from continuous depression and anxiety for many years. He became worse when he developed a cough and weight loss and was told he had lung cancer which 'could not be cured but might be shrivelled up for 12 months or so.' After two cycles of chemotherapy, his physical symptoms had improved and the depression was gone. He said 'I was pleased to be told what was wrong. I couldn't have had better treatment if I'd been a millionaire. If I've only got 12 months they're going to be happy ones.'*

## CLASSIFYING ATTITUDES

One scheme for classifying attitudes, derived from studies of breast cancer patients in London (Greer *et al.*, 1979), consists of four mutually exclusive categories. Like all classification schemes, this one does not always fit the individual case, for some patients show a mixture of more than one attitude at once, and others undergo a change in attitude over time. All the same it provides a useful working basis for studies on this subject, including research into the intriguing possibility that mental attitude is linked with physical prognosis (Section III.3). The four categories are as follows:

1. *Stoic acceptance*: patients show a realistic appreciation of the facts of their illness, and they adopt a calm, fatalistic, and rather passive attitude towards it.
'I just accept it, there's no point getting upset.'
'I'm quite prepared, I've had a good life after all' (she was only 48).
Stoic acceptance is the commonest attitude, and would seem in keeping with the personality traits which are believed to be characteristic of those who develop cancer in the first place (Section I.4).
2. *Helplessness/hopelessness:* patients seem engulfed with despair about their illness and display no initiative in trying to adapt.
'I can't see any future, this seems like the end of the world.'

This attitude may not be a lasting one, but a symptom of clinical depression which could be cured by psychiatric treatment (Section II.7).

3. *Fighting spirit:* patients are determined to master their illness and recover from it.

'Cancer's not going to get me down, don't worry — I've coped with far worse than this.'

Such patients want to take an active part in their own or other people's treatment, and are hungry for information, for example asking to see photographs showing the result of breast surgery before they have their own, reading about their illness and asking lots of questions, and organizing self-help groups.

4. *Denial:* the failure to 'take in' the diagnosis or its implications.
'They haven't said what's wrong, but it's probably nothing much anyway.'

Denial justifies more detailed consideration because it is a term often misused and unfairly condemned. Making value judgements about the merits of different coping styles should be avoided, for different styles suit different patients. Present fashion favours honest exchange of information and open display of feelings. Patients who are reserved, or do not seem sufficiently upset about their illness, are sometimes wrongly criticized for hiding behind the coward's refuge of 'denial'.

The term denial refers to an unconscious mechanism which cannot be demonstrated directly, but may be suspected if a patient fails to ask about diagnosis or prognosis despite ample opportunity: 'forgets' what he has been told: or seems to know the facts in an intellectual sense without showing appropriate distress. Some patients who appear to be using denial are not doing so at all: they are fully aware of the truth but choose not to talk about it. Denial is certainly undesirable in some situations, for example when it leads to long delays in the diagnosis of cancer (Section I.7), prevents patients from complying with treatment, or impedes communication between patients and their relatives, but in other instances it is a valuable defence which helps patients to cope better.

Partial or fluctuating denial is very common: 'My husband died from cancer so I know what it's all about, though in my case I'm confident there's nothing like that, it's merely strain from heavy lifting.' Another example is the patient who knows radiotherapy is used to treat cancer, makes no protest about receiving radiotherapy himself, yet claims to have no idea what is wrong with him. Patients like this evidently realize on one level what is wrong, but denial keeps them unaware of the full gravity of their plight, and so protects them from undue distress. Attempts to force them into stark confrontation with the truth serve no useful purpose.

Lesser degrees of denial merge with the harmless strategy of 'looking on the bright side.' Many of the patients in my study on breast cancer accounted for their ability to adapt to their illness with statements like these:

'Younger women would be more affected.'
'Women with husbands would be more affected.'
'I feel better than before.'
'The growth was sapping my strength.'
'It wasn't very important compared to my husband's death.'
'I was lucky to have treatment early.'
'You've just got to live from day to day.'

Many of these patients also looked on the bright side when they spoke of the possibility of future recurrence of their cancer. Though they had some inkling that this was on the cards, most of them preferred not to know too much about it and were ready to interpret the available evidence in a favourable light, for example assuming they were guaranteed a permanent cure if their initial bone scan was clear. For a few, this mental equilibrium was upset later on by some external reminder of the threat: a TV programme or magazine article about metastatic breast cancer, or hearing that a friend or acquaintance had developed a recurrence of the same disease. Others managed to retain their equilibrium despite such threats: 'I was luckier, mine was caught early.'

An American study on breast cancer (Taylor, 1983) presents a detailed analysis of the mental strategies which enable patients to feel they have gained mastery over their illness. These include concentrating on the positive aspects and ignoring the rest, finding a convincing personal explanation for becoming ill, changing their lifestyle in ways they believed would protect their future health, and comparing themselves favourably with other women who were worse off or had not adapted so well. These strategies combine elements of both 'denial' and 'fighting spirit.'

Patients whose psychological make-up allows them to take comfort from attitudes like these are perhaps more fortunate than those who appreciate the full realities of their condition more clearly.

# 6. Doctor-Patient Communication

Many patients with cancer are ill-informed about their illness. A minority do not know they have cancer at all: others are ignorant of such important aspects as whether their illness is curable and what part treatment will play. The culture of the society in which they live determines to some extent how much they know. American cancer patients, for example, are usually well informed, but in certain European countries with conservative values it is still conventional for a diagnosis of cancer to be withheld from the patient. In Britain, the position is somewhere in between. Cancer is discussed much more openly than it used to be in this country, but there is a wide variation in how much different patients know and how much different doctors consider it right to tell. Some doctors reserve truthful explanations for the patients they think will be able to understand and tolerate them, which usually means the younger, well-educated ones, but ability to cope with cancer is an individual matter, probably depending more on personality than on age or social class.

No single communication policy can be correct for all patients, but research suggests that not being told enough is a more common complaint than being told too much. When problems arise from insufficient communication, the patient is often partly responsible. Patients are often diffident about asking questions and explain this by reasons which appear sound: 'They're always so busy' or 'It's up to them to decide how much they tell you.' These rational statements are often being used to conceal patients' ambivalence about learning truths which might distress them. They fear they will not be able to cope if the news is bad, so consciously or unconsciously they decide it is best not to ask questions. 'Denial' is operating here: the patient probably suspects the truth but in order to avoid intolerable mental distress he makes sure nobody has the opportunity to put his fear into words. An even more striking illustration of denial is seen in those cases where the doctor has talked frankly to the patient about his illness but the patient has completely failed to take it in, and insists he has been told nothing.

Doctors, in their turn, must take a share of the blame for problems in communication. They may fail to take any initiative in telling patients about their illness, fail to give them any clear opportunity to ask questions, and respond to any questions they do ask with euphemisms, evasions, or outright lies. Sometimes this is because the doctor genuinely believes it is in the patient's best interests to remain in ignorance. This may be correct in some cases, for example for an elderly patient who would not have long to live anyway and regards cancer as carrying a strong stigma. Often, however, the doctor cannot know how the patient would in fact react given the opportunity, and is using the excuse of protecting the patient when his real intention is to shield himself from the difficult task of imparting bad news.

Unconfirmed suspicions about having cancer are more stressful for many patients than definite knowledge of the diagnosis. Some patients who have been devastated by unspoken fears are able to 'rally round' when they know the real facts and are able to talk openly about their condition. Conversely, patients who through ignorance and denial were quite unprepared for hearing their diagnosis may 'go to pieces' if it is revealed to them too suddenly or, worse still, if they learn it by accident.

## STUDIES OF PATIENTS' SATISFACTION WITH COMMUNICATION

One of the first systematic studies in this field (Aitken-Swan and Easson, 1959) was carried out at a time when cancer patients in Britain were seldom informed of their diagnosis, and only fatal cases of cancer were likely to come to public notice. The intention of the study was to publicize the fact that some cancers are curable, in the hope that this would lessen the dread which surrounded the disease, and encourage other patients to present early for treatment. To this end, 231 new patients whose cancers were judged to have an excellent prognosis were told their diagnosis by their consultant. During later follow-up interviews, the patients' reactions to this knowledge were gauged. The majority, 153 patients, approved of having been told: 44 denied the knowledge: 17 (all women) disapproved: and in 17 cases the reaction could not be classified. For 35 cases, the GP's opinion was also sought, and all 35 approved of their patients being told, often commenting they had taken the news well and their management was much easier. Nearly thirty years later, frank disclosure of the diagnosis to patients with curable cancers is common, though not universal, medical policy.

A group of patients with Hodgkin's disease or other lymphomas, potentially curable conditions, were studied in Edinburgh (Lloyd *et al.,* 1984). They all knew their diagnosis, and all approved of having been told. Eleven of 31 patients, however, were dissatisfied with one or more aspects of communication: they reported inadequate information about the illness, inadequate information about the treatment, and/or insufficient time to ask questions of staff. The patients who said they were dissatisfied with communication had obtained higher neuroticism scores on the initial personality assessment than the rest, but they did not differ regarding their levels of depression or anxiety.

In contrast many lung cancer patients, who have a far worse prognosis, apparently prefer not to have too much information spelled out. When they first came to hospital, 183 English patients with inoperable lung cancer (Jones, 1981) were told they would be having investigations to detect various named diseases, including cancer. They were also told they would be given a truthful answer if they chose to ask about their diagnosis after these tests were complete, but that if they did not ask, the information would only be given to their GPs.

Ninety patients did ask; only one subsequently objected to being told but ten seemed to 'deny' the knowledge. Ninety-three never asked, but 42 of them spoke in ways which suggested they knew they had a fatal disease.

Table 4. Responses of 62 lung cancer patients to questions on knowledge of diagnosis and prognosis and satisfaction with information given

| | |
|---|---:|
| 1. Knowledge of diagnosis | |
| Knew the diagnosis of cancer and were well-informed about the details | 15 |
| Knew the diagnosis of cancer but no more | 28 |
| Suspected cancer but had not been told | 9 |
| Appeared completely ignorant, or misinformed | 10 |
| 2. Knowledge of prognosis | |
| Fully confident of recovery | 15 |
| Hoping to recover but aware they might not | 14 |
| Knew they were likely to die quite soon | 20 |
| Don't know or vague reply | 13 |
| 3. Satisfaction with information from doctors | |
| Satisfied (and aware of the diagnosis) | 33 |
| Satisfied (but seemed poorly informed) | 13 |
| Not satisfied (not told enough) | 16 |
| Not satisfied (told too much) | 0 |

In my own study of lung cancer, questions on knowledge of diagnosis and prognosis, and satisfaction with information given by doctors, were put to 62 patients about three months after the diagnosis had been made. A classification of their replies is given in Table 4, but actual quotations give a more vivid impression of the wide variation which was found, and the frequency of changing or ambivalent attitudes:

'First of all they didn't tell me anything and I was a little bit agitated. Then I asked straight out if I'd got cancer and I felt 100% better when they told me.'

'I never question them at all. What you don't know you can't worry about, can you?'

'I don't believe it's my business to question them, because I don't understand the medical side.'

'I'd have liked to ask a few more questions but you don't like to ask too many, with all those others queuing up outside. And I'd like to see the consultant again — but you get a different understudy every time.'

'I know what I've got, so I don't ask questions.'

'They told my daughter it could be cancer but I don't believe it, because I feel so well.'

'Do you know, they've lost the path results, so they can't tell me a thing' (the biopsy report of cancer was in fact filed in her casenotes).

'I'm starting special treatment for this lung cancer. I didn't really take in what they said about it — couldn't remember a thing afterwards — though I doubt very much they've got a cure.'

'I get the impression it can't be cured, but can be checked, from the reading I've done. The doctors don't say a thing — I admire the way they can guard you off. I'd like to know my prognosis, so I can make arrangements.'

'They didn't say a thing to me but they told my daughter it was cancer, and she told me.'

'I know there's no cure, but I hope these injections will put a few years on my life. I consider it a bonus these doctors have answered my questions so frankly.'

Breast cancer, in contrast to some other types of cancer, is so well-publicized that it must be difficult for any patient nowadays to remain in ignorance of having the condition, however little individual doctor-patient communication exists and however prone to denial the patient may be. However, a few of the 44 breast cancer patients I followed up after mastectomy did seem to be in doubt about what was wrong, for example the woman who remarked six months later 'They've never said whether it was cancer, but I suppose it must have been.' Others, though fully aware they had cancer, expressed diffidence about asking for details: 'I didn't like to ask why I had to have chemotherapy', 'I was too scared to ask if it was a bad cancer.' Many patients stressed how desirable it was to be able to see the same doctor every time they attended the follow-up clinic.

## SUMMARY

Many cancer patients in Britain are badly informed about their illness, partly due to doctors' failure to give them information, partly due to their own reluctance to ask questions or accept what they have been told. Some patients are able to cope better if they do not know too much, others are distressed about barriers to communication. Cancer patients who are well-informed, on the other hand, seldom complain of being told too much. Patients with curable forms of cancer are naturally more likely to welcome information than patients whose cancer has a poor prognosis.

# 7. Depression in Cancer Patients

## INTRODUCTION

Depressive illness, depression for short, is a very common mental disorder in which the essential feature is lowering of mood. In cancer patients, depression is even more common than it is in the population as a whole, but many cases are never recognized. This is regrettable, because effective treatments are available. A general review of depression and its management in cancer patients is given by Goldberg (1981).

## SYMPTOMS

The symptoms of depression can conveniently be divided into two groups, mental and physical. Mental symptoms include sadness, loss of interest, inability to concentrate, irritablity, guilt, low self-esteem, pessimism, and thoughts of suicide. Some depressed patients are acutely aware of their misery and can express this by weeping: others simply complain of feeling empty or slowed down, and cannot cry even if they believe tears would bring relief. Anxiety and agitation are mixed with depression in some cases. Physical symptoms include loss of appetite and weight (less often gain), insomnia (less often excessive sleep), constipation, tiredness, loss of energy, reduced activity, impotence in men, and loss of sexual interest in women, a general feeling of malaise, headaches, or other types of pain in various body parts. Some patients show a 'diurnal variation' which can be a useful pointer to the diagnosis: they wake early and feel at their worst in the mornings, but gradually improve towards the end of each day.

In cancer patients, the physical symptoms are not very helpful in deciding whether depression is present, because they are so similar to the symptoms of cancer itself. Diagnosis relies much more on the mental symptoms.

## DIAGNOSIS

There is no clear-cut distinction between depressive illness, or 'clinical depression', and the 'normal' depression of mood, or 'depressive reaction', which most people experience in distressing circumstances. This distinction is especially difficult in cancer patients, who have such obvious reason to feel depressed. Many cancer patients go through a depressive reaction, lasting a few days or weeks, at some stage during their illness and this is often considered a natural part of the process of acceptance and adjustment. Depressive illnesses, on the other hand, do not serve any useful function, but merely add greatly to patients' suffering. For research purposes it is essential to draw a fixed dividing line between patients who are depressed and those who are not by applying a standard set of criteria, for example those given in the 'DSM III' (American Psychiatric Association, 1980).

In clinical practice, depressive illness should be considered if a patient's depressed mood seems much more severe or long-lasting than that which most patients show in similar circumstances, or if he expresses unduly morbid ideas, for example regarding himself as a worthless burden whose existence holds no pleasure or purpose. Such attitudes are neither usual nor justified in cancer patients, who usually retain an intact sense of self-esteem and continue to appreciate their relationships with others, however grim their physical state may be. Clinical depression is reasonably easy to recognize so long as the possibility is kept in mind. A miserable expression, despondent manner or a neglected appearance are common clues, though some depressed patients present a smiling front. Tactful unhurried inquiry about how patients feel in their spirits, or how they think they are coping with their illness, provides the opportunity for depressive symptoms, or other psychological difficulties, to be revealed. One simple way to screen patients for the presence of a mood disorder is to ask them to complete a questionnaire: a good example is the Hospital Anxiety and Depression Scale or HAD (Zigmond and Snaith, 1983), in which all the items are concerned with mental and not physical symptoms.

## CAUSES

Depression in patients with cancer may result from three broad factors (Table 5): psychological reactions to the illness or its treatment, physical effects of the illness or its treatment on the brain, and reasons unconnected with the illness. Several different factors are often operating together in the same patient, and it is seldom possible to isolate one single cause in any individual case.

Table 5. Causes of depression in cancer patients

---

1. Reactive to the stress of the illness:
   Physical symptoms, e.g. pain, weakness, breathlessness
   Knowledge of a poor prognosis, and/or stigma of 'cancer'
   Side-effects of treatment, e.g. disfiguring surgery, nausea from radiotherapy or cytotoxic drugs

2. Organic brain syndromes:
   Cerebral metastases
   Metabolic impairments, e.g. hypercalcaemia, liver failure, ectopic hormone secretion
   Drug effects, e.g. steroids (though euphoria is a more common effect), cytotoxics

3. Chance association in patients with:
   Past history of depression
   Family history of depression
   Other recent 'life events' or social problems

---

Cancer patients with a previous history of depression, neurotic personality traits, and unhappy social circumstances are all at increased risk of depression. If the physical symptoms of the cancer are severe, or if the patient knows that the physical prognosis is bad, depression is again more likely. Some kinds of treatment for cancer are more likely to give rise to depression than others. Awareness of these associations helps doctors to be more alert to the likelihood of depression developing in especially vulnerable groups of patients, but it is no substitute for individual assessment of each case.

## FREQUENCY

Depression is the most common mental disorder among whole populations of cancer patients and also among the minority who are referred to psychiatrists. The main diagnoses for 50 hospitalized cancer patients referred for psychiatric consultation in London (Hinton, 1972) were as follows: depression 28 cases, anxiety state 14 cases, confusional state 5 cases, phobic state 2 cases, and personality disorder 1 case.

As there is no clearcut definition of 'depression', and 'cancer' includes a wide variety of diseases, the question 'What proportion of cancer patients are depressed?' can have no precise answer. But taking round figures from a number of different studies, a reasonable generalization would be that for any population of cancer patients at any one time up to 25% have severe or moderate depression, another 25% have mild depression, and about 50% are not depressed at all. Four American studies on patients with cancer of mixed types (Plumb and Holland, 1977; Craig and Abeloff, 1974; Derogatis *et al.*, 1983; Bukberg *et al.*, 1984) have found the prevalence of depression to be of this order.

An indirect way to study the frequency of severe depression in cancer patients is to examine their suicide rates. A records study of this kind was carried out in Connecticut (Fox *et al.*, 1982) for a huge sample of patients officially registered as having cancer. A two-fold increase over general population suicide rates was found for the men, but not the women. Even if some cases of suicide in patients already suffering from advanced cancer go undetected, or unreported, suicide in such patients is clearly not a frequent event.

Patients with early breast cancer have been the subject of many psychological studies (for example Morris *et al.*, 1977; Maguire *et al.*, 1978). These show that about a third of patients have an episode of depression and/or anxiety in the year following diagnosis. The type of treatment given influences the risk of depression: patients given adjuvant chemotherapy after mastectomy are more likely to become depressed than those treated by mastectomy alone (Maguire *et al.*, 1980), and patients who have a mastectomy may be more likely to become depressed than those who have 'lumpectomy' (Steinburg *et al.*, 1985), though further research is required to settle this question. In my own series of breast cancer patients followed up after mastectomy, 14 of 44 (32%) had an episode of depression, but only in eight cases was this both profound and prolonged. For some, the depression seemed to be mainly reactive to the loss of the breast, and for others, fear of recurrent cancer was apparently the cause: a few attributed their depression to other social problems not connected with the cancer.

A sample of lymphoma patients was followed through treatment with radiotherapy and/or chemotherapy in Edinburgh (Lloyd *et al.*, 1984). Depression and/or anxiety was found in 14 out of 40 patients a fortnight after diagnosis, and in eight of the 31 interviewed after treatment was finished.

I studied the frequency and apparent causes of depression in a series of 138 lung cancer patients interviewed at the time of presentation to hospital. Severe or 'major' depression was present in 19 (14%), and mild or 'minor' depression in another 30 (22%), a total of 49 (36%). About a third of the depressed patients thought their depression was due to the fear of having cancer: another third thought the main reason was inability to continue their usual activities because of a physical symptom like breathlessness or pain; and the remaining third related their depression to some other event like a recent bereavement. The presence of major depression was found to have statistical associations with the following factors: spread of tumour beyond the chest, oat cell histological type, physical dependency, a past history of depression, and the experience of certain other defined 'life events' in the past two years. Severe depression was more frequent among the men, though in the general population, women are more likely to become depressed.

About three months after diagnosis, interviews with 62 lung cancer patients (many of the original sample had already died, or were too ill to be interviewed) showed major depression in 10 cases (16%) and minor depression in 21 (43%). None of the patients who had had surgical treatment with the aim of cure were depressed, and the most severe and profound depressions were found among patients who had not received any specific treatment at all. Again, physically dependent patients were most likely to be depressed. Reasons which the patients themselves gave to explain their depression included (in order of frequency): feeling so ill, the side-effects of chemotherapy, the prospect of death, being unable to do things, loneliness, uncertainty about what was wrong or what was going to happen, pain, the side-effects of radiotherapy, worry about dependent relatives, and feeling not enough was being done. Failure of doctor-communication was a prominent feature in their complaints, though it was often difficult to say whether this was a cause or an effect of the depression.

A selection of case histories follows.

1. *A married man in his 70's, who had been depressed on and off since having pneumonia four years beforehand, presented with a persistent cough. His chest X-ray was suspicious of lung cancer but the bronchoscopy failed to prove the diagnosis. At follow-up he was so weak his wife had to help him bath and dress, and he had chest pain which was not controlled by analgesic tablets. He was profoundly miserable and very irritable. His GP had just started him on an antidepressant (amitriptyline). He said 'They say it could be malignant, but I'd be too old for major surgery. By the time I go back to the hospital I'm afraid it'll be too late, I'm going downhill so fast.' (Shortly after this he was readmitted and tests confirmed lung cancer, but he died soon afterwards.)*

2. *A married man in his 70's had been disabled by arterial disease of the legs for ten years. He then developed difficulty in swallowing and lost weight. He had been told he had a shadow on the lung, and said 'If it is cancer, I've asked the doctor to let me know.' He had been depressed for some years and thought this was partly due to the pain in his legs, partly to worry about his invalid wife. He was taking an antidepressant (mianserin). Investigations confirmed lung cancer, but the symptoms were not considered severe enough to merit palliative radiotherapy. At follow-up he said 'I've no idea what they found. I'm eating better, but my breathing worries me. My doctor just says it will improve.' He was more depressed than ever, and kept having crying spells, but did not know why.*

3. *A married man in his 50's kept getting chest infections. He knew there was a shadow on his lung and was afraid it was cancer, but was too scared to ask, and after the diagnosis was confirmed he was not told at first. He had a course of palliative radiotherapy, which he found 'eerie and frightening,' but admitted that it had 'done a tremendous job' in improving his symptoms. He became both depressed and anxious when he 'couldn't get a straight answer' about what was wrong. Eventually one of his doctors confirmed he had cancer, but his worries about his prognosis were not discussed, and he remained 'on edge' and unable to sleep. It was several weeks before the word 'cancer' could be spoken between him and his wife. She herself was even more depressed than her husband, feeling so stigmatized by his diagnosis that she dared not go out shopping and describing the recent events as 'one long nightmare.'*

4. *A married man in his 80's developed a persistent cough. Though superficially cheerful, and remarkably alert for his age, he admitted on direct questioning to many depressive symptoms, which he put down to worry about his frail blind wife. Bronchoscopy demonstrated a tumour and he received a course of radiotherapy. He became weepy following each treatment, but had no other side-effects, and considered the*

*radiotherapy well worthwhile because his cough had improved. Although he had not been told his diagnosis, he had privately come to the conclusion that he had incurable cancer and 'had better make arrrangements.' His wife had coped far better than he expected. His depressive symptoms were worse but he could not pinpoint a reason.*

*5. A married man in his 50's had four months' history of breathlessness, chest pain, and weakness. He became deeply depressed in reaction to his forced inactivity and worry about cancer. The diagnosis of cancer was confirmed, and he was told of this. Chemotherapy was started but the tumour did not respond, and at the time of followup he was impatiently awaiting a course of radiotherapy. He was prepared to have any treatment, however drastic, if it would retard the progression of his disease. He was still depressed: 'I suppose it's fear of the future . . . I've laid out my affairs so my wife will know what to do . . . it's not particularly pleasant.' His wife had herself been very upset, but was supportive, and their relationship had grown closer.*

*6. A married man in his 60's had had chronic bronchitis for years. He had also received psychiatric treatment for depression and alcoholism. When admitted for investigation of increasing breathlessness, he was depressed again and put this down to the inactivity enforced by his physical state. Lung cancer was diagnosed, and treated by radiotherapy. He was physically weak, and continuously tearful, while this treatment was in progress, but after it finished his breathing improved 'like a miracle.' It was not clear whether he knew his diagnosis: 'What you don't know you can't worry about, can you.' He continued to have bouts of deeply depressed mood which he could not explain. His wife said she felt desperate, having to cope with him when he was such a misery, and being unable to afford to go out for any diversions.*

*7. A man of 70 presented with cough and chest pain, three weeks after his wife had died. He was depressed over her loss. X-rays suggested a tumour but bronchoscopy was negative, and no treatment was given. At follow-up he was getting a lot*

*of pain in his ribs and said 'I get more useless every week.'
He guessed he had cancer, though 'The doctors have said
nothing. They've got too many to see — they don't know or
care about you as an individual. I don't mind if they tell me
or not, it's up to them. I'm in the final chapter of my life, I
believe — and hope.'* He considered that loneliness was the
main reason for his continuing depression.

## MANAGEMENT

Many cases of depression in patients with cancer are not
recognized by medical staff. Depressed patients often make no
direct complaint about their symptoms, because the depression
makes them regard themselves as a nuisance or a burden whose
case is hopeless anyway. Such patients would usually admit how
they feel in response to tactful questioning but may not get the
opportunity, because many doctors have a well-meaning
reluctance to ask about emotional problems in cancer patients:
they are afraid their questions will merely upset both the
patients and themselves, by drawing attention to distress for
which no remedy is available. This is a misguided attitude. A
useful analogy may be drawn between depression and pain:
both common symptoms of cancer which can and should be
controlled by appropriate treatment. Depressed cancer patients
often feel better simply for talking about their problems to
someone who can understand, and if this is not enough they
often respond to one or more of the measures outlined below.

### Treating organic brain syndromes

An important first step is to identify, and if possible correct,
any physical pathology which might be contributing to the
depression. A depressed patient with cerebral metastases, for
example, would probably improve mentally after a course of
radiotherapy to the brain, but might merely develop a
confusional state if given antidepressant drugs. Similarly,

metabolic and hormonal disturbances giving rise to depression are best corrected directly when this is possible. Some doctors think of depression in purely psychological terms and forget it may be due to organic brain disturbance: in a report on 100 cancer patients referred to a psychiatrist in an American centre (Levine *et al.,* 1978), 40 had organic brain syndromes which had usually been missed.

## Improving Communication

Inadequate understanding of the illness, or difficulty in being able to talk about it with either doctors or close relatives, often accompany depression, and an attempt to improve communication problems should be an early priority. Simply giving patient and relative, perhaps together, clear opportunities to ask questions or express their worries in a private unhurried setting, may lead to marked improvements in mood for them both. Sometimes communication problems cannot be solved so easily, however: patient and relatives may resist being drawn into discussion, especially if the patient is so depressed as to be totally absorbed in guilt and despair, and in a few cases a patient becomes even more depressed when the truth about his illness is confirmed.

## Antidepressant drugs

(Crammer *et al.,* 1982): these include tricyclic compounds like amitriptyline and imipramine, newer drugs such as mianserin, and the monoamine oxidase inhibitors (MAOI's) such as phenelzine. Drugs are effective for about 70% of depressed patients in general psychiatric practice, but the proportion of depressed cancer patients who respond well to these drugs is not known. There may be a delay of two to six weeks before improvement becomes apparent, and an effective drug should be continued several months more to prevent relapse. The common side-effects are dry mouth, drowsiness, and faintness on standing due to a lowering of blood pressure: all these diminish as the body gets used to the drug. If one drug does not help, a different one may be more effective.

**Psychotherapy**

Many different techniques are covered by the term 'psychotherapy' (Brown and Pedder, 1979; Storr, 1979), but they all involve approaching emotional difficulties through exchange of words in the setting of a professional relationship. This may be done either individually or in small groups. Psychotherapy is more than just talking over problems, since it requires the patient to face up to unacknowledged aspects of his feelings and behaviour, and to take responsibility for making emotional changes. Formal psychoanalysis is a prolonged, intensive and arduous treatment which few cancer patients would be robust enough to complete, and is not usually suitable for treating depression in any case. Other more modern types of psychotherapy, however, are sometimes appropriate in this setting. Two examples are 'brief focal psychotherapy' (Malan, 1979), in which techniques derived from psychoanalysis are applied to a specific problem in a limited number of sessions: and 'cognitive therapy' (Mackay, 1982) which entails identifying depressed patients' unjustified negative thoughts and beliefs, and encouraging them to replace these by positive ones. Cancer patients who are to benefit from any form of psychotherapy need to be reasonably well informed about their diagnosis and prognosis.

**Electroconvulsive therapy (ECT)**

ECT (Kendell, 1981) is a safe and rapidly acting treatment for depression, generally reserved for the most severe cases in which it works best. ECT involves the passage of a small electric current across the brain while the patient is under a short-acting anaesthetic. In the undrugged patient such a current would cause an epileptic fit, but a muscle relaxant is given to reduce the fit to a slight twitching. ECT is given two or three times a week and several treatments, usually about six, are needed to relieve depression. The only common side-effect is memory loss, which recovers after a few weeks. ECT is often assumed to be too drastic a treatment for cancer patients but this is not logical, unless the patient is too ill to withstand the anaesthetic.

There are no firm rules about which combination of these treatments should be used, or in what order. Mild cases of depression often clear up with counselling alone, or counselling plus a course of antidepressant drugs given by the GP or cancer treatment specialist. Severe or resistant cases of depression should be referred to a psychiatrist who, depending on the nature of the symptoms, may recommend a change of drug, a course of psychotherapy, or a course of ECT.

Depression preceding a diagnosis of cancer is considered in Section I.3, and depression among terminally ill patients in Section III.1.

## SUMMARY

Surveys show that a substantial minority of patients with cancer develop clinical depression of a severity which merits treatment. This may be a psychological reaction to the stress of the illness and/or a reflection of disordered brain function caused by physical complications of the illness. Many cases of depression are either not recognized or not treated, although the majority would improve with a combination of counselling and an antidepressant drug. A few depressed cancer patients need psychiatric referral for consideration of psychotherapy or ECT.

# 8. Counselling

Counselling programmes for cancer patients aim to improve both physical and mental welfare. They include providing practical information about the illness and its treatment, and giving patients the opportunity to express and discuss their feelings. Since counselling is designed to encourage optimum adjustment for everyone, rather than being a treatment for problems already present, programmes are usually intended for all patients and not just those who are coping badly. Counselling may be carried out either individually or in small groups.

## WHO PROVIDES COUNSELLING?

Hospital medical staff and GPs often provide a certain amount of counselling as an integral part of their cancer patients' treatment, and thus succeed in meeting their emotional needs as well as caring for them physically. This is not always so: some doctors and nurses who excel in the practical aspects of their work do not have the interest or skills to tackle psychological problems, and even if they do, they seldom have time to provide this service for all their patients. Sometimes, perhaps for fear of appearing ungrateful, patients find it easier to reveal worries or problems to someone who is not directly concerned with their physical treatment.

Some cancer treatment units have a staff member who specializes in counselling. Often this is a nurse with special knowledge of a certain condition, for example several units in Britain now employ mastectomy nurses who take a routine part in the management of breast cancer patients. These nurses provide guidance on the choice of prosthesis and other aspects of physical rehabilitation, at the same time as monitoring their patients for depression, anxiety or sexual problems which may need treatment. The widespread appreciation of the service provided by one such nursing sister in Southampton is evident from many breast cancer patients' comments. Similar services are not so widely available after other cancer operations such as colostomy or laryngectomy, though they would be equally valuable. Social workers may be the best group of professionals to provide counselling on aspects not concerned with physical care, especially the emotional and practical problems which may affect a whole family when one member has cancer.

Other patients who have received treatment for the same form of cancer in the past sometimes prove more effective or more acceptable counsellors than professional staff. Self-help groups run by volunteers reflect this. Most of them can arrange individual counselling as well as group meetings.

Some patients, of course, prefer to discuss their difficulties with someone who has no specialized knowledge about cancer, for example with clergy or close friends.

## DRAWBACKS OF COUNSELLING PROGRAMMES

Though counselling is welcomed by many patients, and its benefits might seem to be obvious, it has potential negative aspects as well. Many cancer patients have no need for professional counselling, because they have sufficient personality resources and family supports to enable them to adjust to their illness by themselves. Counselling for such patients is a luxury, and not a wise use of scarce health service time or money. Not all cancer patients accept counselling when it is offered and the patients who would seem likely to benefit most are often the ones who refuse, because they are ashamed of their problems, or find it difficult to talk about them.

Counselling involves patients being reasonably well-informed about their illness, whereas some patients would cope better by using denial, only knowing as much as they can accept.

In a group setting, for example, patients may be upset by learning of recurrences or deaths in other group members and start worrying about their own prognosis.

Counsellors without adequate medical knowledge may miss certain mental or physical problems altogether, or else make a misguided attempt to manage these themselves. Severe depression, for example, will not respond to counselling alone, but requires treatment with drugs or ECT. A few lay counsellors have taken up the work from unsuitable motives and their interventions are harmful: they may deliberately turn their clients against conventional medical treatments in favour of useless 'alternative therapies', or they may unconsciously be seeking help for their own difficulties and possess no expertise in helping to solve other people's problems.

For these reasons, it is important for counselling programmes to be evaluated by an objective observer before they are widely introduced on the intuitive assumption that they must be a good thing.

## EVALUATING COUNSELLING PROGRAMMES

I will describe two American studies designed to evaluate counselling programmes for cancer patients. A wider-ranging review of the findings of such studies is provided by Watson (1983).

The first study, from New York, was concerned with individual counselling (Gordon *et al.*, 1980). All new patients with lung cancer, breast cancer or melanoma admitted to a certain hospital over a certain time period were asked to take part; patients with the same diagnoses admitted over a different time period formed a control group, making a total of about 300 patients. Each patient in the first group was allocated to an 'oncology counsellor' trained in psychology, social work or psychiatric nursing, who would see the patient every day during the hospital admission then as often as seemed necessary following discharge. The counsellor provided education about cancer and its treatment, and discussed psychological aspects, and would refer patients to specialized agencies as required. Both counselled and control groups were assessed, on four occasions during one year, by an independent person. The findings were that about 20% of patients offered counselling refused it from the start, and about 12% who began the counselling dropped out later on. Those who did complete the counselling programme, however, were found to have a better adjustment than the controls in some respects, including better solving of problems, more rapid decline of negative mood, more realistic outlook on life, and greater likelihood of returning to work. No unwanted effects were reported.

The second study, from California, was concerned with group counselling (Spiegel *et al.*, 1981). Eighty-six women with metastatic breast cancer whose oncologists considered them suitable for the study (that is, an already selected sample) were randomly assigned to attend a group or to form a control. Each group consisted of 7-10 patients and had two leaders, one a psychiatrist or social worker, the other a patient who had been successfully treated for breast cancer in the past. They met each week for 90 minutes. The group was designed to share problems and provide mutual support, but deep analysis or challenging confrontation was not encouraged. The patients were assessed with a battery of psychological tests every four months for a year. Only 30 of the original 86 patients completed the study, due to a mixture of dropouts and deaths. Compared to the controls, patients who took part in group therapy were better adjusted on some of the outcome measures, but no different on others. Group members reported improved relationships with their doctors, less sense of isolation, and greater ability to face death. The deaths of other patients in the group were distressing, but ultimately viewed as having enhanced the remaining patients' experience. No major unwanted effects were reported.

## SUMMARY

Formal counselling is welcomed by many patients as a means of helping them adjust to having cancer. Counselling carried out by properly trained staff has been found to bring benefits with few unwanted effects, though counselling by untrained volunteers may cause distress. Some patients do not want counselling, or do not need it.

# 9. The Relatives

When one member of a family has cancer, the mental suffering of the healthy relatives may be at least as great as that of the patient himself. Husbands, wives, parents, and children each have their own special problems.

Relatives in this situation often feel obliged to present a brave face, especially if they have had to take over practical tasks and responsibilities from the patient. They are afraid that revealing their own distress will upset the patient and make him feel a burden, or make them appear selfishly absorbed in their own problems instead of putting the patient's welfare first. Therefore they hesitate to seek help on their own account.

Problems of a rather opposite kind can arise when relatives are prevented from enjoying any activities of their own for fear of appearing frivolous or callous, or seeming to wish the patient out of the way. This is especially likely if they want to continue some formerly shared hobby which the patient is no longer well enough to take part in, or make plans for their own future in which the patient is not involved. When patients and relatives are both afraid of upsetting each other, they often avoid discussing the illness at all, and become emotionally estranged.

The medical practice of revealing a cancer diagnosis to a relative but not telling the patient is still favoured by some doctors, though it seems difficult to justify unless the patient is too young, too old or too ill to understand the situation. Except for patients of this kind, the practice seems to breach the rules of doctor-patient confidentiality, and often imposes a heavy burden on the relative. Sometimes it is relatives and not doctors who decide this course is best:

*A woman whose husband was found to have lung cancer was determined he should not be told. Each time he attended hospital for chemotherapy, she asked to see the doctor first to remind him not to mention the diagnosis. One day she did not manage to do this, and a new doctor casually mentioned 'cancer' to the patient, assuming he would already know what was wrong. The patient, an inarticulate man who had been rather puzzled and unhappy till that point, said he was very pleased to know. After that, the couple were able to talk to each other much more easily, and the wife admitted it was a big relief.*

## SURVEYS OF DEPRESSION AND ANXIETY AMONG RELATIVES

An estimate of the frequency of clinical depression among relatives can be made from an American study about depression in hospitalized cancer patients (Plumb and Holland, 1977) which used patients' spouses or parents as one of the control groups. Of 66 relatives, 18% scored in the 'moderately depressed' range of the assessment scale, but none scored as severely depressed. When only the psychological symptoms of depression were considered, depression was equally common among the patients and their relatives.

About 200 cancer outpatients and their next-of-kin were studied by means of mood questionnaires in another American study (Cassileth *et al.,* 1985a). The patients as a group were found to have rather more mood disturbance than the relatives, but there was a correlation between the scores for patient-relative pairs: that is, if a patient reported a high degree of anxiety or depression, his relative was likely to do so too. For both patients and relatives, anxiety and depression were most common while treatment was in progress, or when the cancer had reached an advanced stage, and least common when patients were on follow-up during periods of remission.

## HUSBANDS AND WIVES

Development of cancer in one partner may either strengthen or weaken a marriage relationship. If the relationship was previously a good one, it usually withstands the pressures of the illness and may even grow closer as a result. Previously shaky marriages may break down completely under the strain, but sometimes they too become better during the course of the illness.

Of the 39 married lung cancer patients I interviewed about three months after diagnosis, all but three said they had received emotional support from their spouse, of whom they often spoke with admiration and praise. About half the group, however, were aware that the spouse was distressed at the same time:
'She must be worn out, but she'd never show it.'
'She's got very poorly and run down — she keeps worrying about me and my cough keeps her awake.'
The remaining three patients considered their spouse too upset too provide any support at all:
'I've tried to make him realize what I've got but he won't listen. The one time I did get through, he broke right down. I don't know how he's going to cope when I've gone.'

No patient perceived any hostility or lack of concern from their spouse, and any problems which had arisen usually concerned couples' ability to communicate regarding the illness. Three of the 27 married patients who were themselves well informed never spoke about their diagnosis for fear of upsetting their spouse, and many others had had problems at first:
'I couldn't tell the wife what the doctor said, my sister had to do it. But the wife reacted 100% better than I expected.'
This study did not include systematic separate interviews with the spouses themselves. Sometimes, when talking to a couple together or briefly seeing the spouse alone, I had the impression that the spouse was far more distressed than the patient seemed to realize.

Of the 28 married patients with breast cancer I followed up after mastectomy, three reported problems had arisen in their marriages but the rest said the relationship was just the same, or even closer. Some data about the marital relationships of patients with terminal cancer is given in Section III.1.

## PARENTS OF CHILDREN WITH CANCER

Most studies involving direct interviews with relatives, as opposed to reports given by patients, have been carried out on the parents of children treated for leukaemia or other types of cancer.

Twenty-four families in which a child with cancer had been successfully treated in a Liverpool hospital were studied some years later (Peck, 1979). None of the parents believed their child was cured and the continuing anxiety 'hung like a cloud over every family.' Six parents' marriages had broken down, usually because the child's illness had put extra strain on an already fragile relationship. Quotations given include:
'He refused to acknowledge that she was ever ill.'
'We both looked to our parents to help us, rather than to each other . . . we blamed each other for the illness.'
'He took refuge in alcohol.'
'I only lived for the child, it didn't matter about anyone else.'
'He just couldn't take the extra responsibility.'

However, six other couples had been brought closer together, and the remaining 12 marriages were apparently unaffected. Half the families would have liked more information about the illness, and almost all emphasized the need to be able to talk to an informed outsider in the period following diagnosis. Less than half the children had been told their diagnosis, and in a third of families there was inhibited communication between parents and children regarding health topics. When there were other children in the family, the siblings sometimes felt jealous of the extra attention given to the sick child, and rejected by their parents, and might develop behavioural problems or 'psychosomatic' symptoms. The doctor was usually named as the main source of help and support, and the desirability of continuing to see the same doctor and nurse throughout hospital treatment was emphasized. About half the families had needed financial help, usually provided from charitable funds, to meet the expenses such as fares to hospital and extra heating imposed by the illness. Following this study, the hospital obtained more social workers to help alleviate the communication difficulties and practical problems which such families experience.

In a more recent study carried out in Manchester (Maguire, 1984), 60 families in which a child was diagnosed as having leukaemia were followed up for 12-18 months by means of a structured psychiatric interview, the Present State Examination (Wing *et al.,* 1974). Depressive illness was present in 27% of mothers, and an anxiety state in 30%, six weeks after the diagnosis, and depression and anxiety were still nearly as common by the end of the study, often both present together in the same mothers. Depression and anxiety were far less common in the control group of families in which a child had been hospitalized for more minor physical illness. Fathers were 'also at risk but less so than the mothers'.

The same paper contains a review of prevention, detection, and treatment of psychiatric disorders and social problems among the families of children with cancer. These problems often go undetected in ordinary clinical practice, because the child's health takes priority, or because staff are reluctant to ask questions which might provoke distress. Visits from a specialized nurse are welcomed by most families, but there is no evidence that this service can actually reduce the frequency of psychosocial problems. Support groups based in the hospital, and self-help groups run by volunteers, require more evaluation. They have advantages, for example reducing the sense of isolation, providing mutual support, and sharing information, but also disadvantages, for example inappropriate advice from under-trained volunteer personnel, and unjustified generalizations stemming from the inclusion of cases with different prognoses. Training in interview skills or the use of screening questionnaires might enable better detection of psychiatric symptoms so that early treatment could be given, though once again there is a need for scientific evaluation of how effective such treatment is.

## SUMMARY

Depression and anxiety among the relatives of cancer patients are probably just as common as among patients themselves, but are less likely to be reported. Most cancer patients consider their relatives a source of emotional support, and families in which one member has cancer often become closer than before, although sometimes the opposite happens.

# PART III: THE FINAL OUTCOME: DEATH OR LONG-TERM SURVIVAL

# 1. Terminal Cancer and its Aftermath

Patients with cancers too advanced for cure eventually reach the terminal phase, when death will inevitably follow within a matter of weeks. The emotional problems affecting terminal patients, and the sources of support which enable them to cope, overlap considerably with those which apply to cancer patients in general and have already been discussed in Part II of this book: the same topics will be more briefly reconsidered here in relation to the terminal phase.

For terminal patients, emotional adjustment can be harder because there is no realistic hope of recovery, and because most patients suffer various unpleasant physical symptoms in addition to being generally weak and helpless. On the other hand some patients, by the time they become terminal, have succeeded in 'working through' the emotional problems of the earlier part of their illness to reach a stage of acceptance: and for others emotional distress is rendered less acute because the pain-relieving drugs they need, or the effect of the illness itself on their brain, is clouding their consciousness and making them less aware of their plight.

Most of the work quoted in this section was done on the selected minority of terminal cancer patients who are admitted to hospices or continuing care units, in which staff have developed special expertise in both physical and psychological aspects of caring for the dying. Other cancer patients die in general hospitals or at home, where the balance of problems and compensations may be rather different.

Our own interview study on 50 consecutive patients admitted to the continuing care unit in Southampton included the question 'What do you think has been the worst part of this illness?' The forced inactivity resulting from a weakened physical state was by far the commonest answer, being given by half the patients. Problems stemming from this forced inactivity included being unable to look after the family, having to watch while other people carried out the patients' former tasks (often not to the patients' satisfaction), and fear of being a burden. Less common worst aspects were specific symptoms like vomiting, pain, or swollen abdomen, being ill and in hospital, fear of death, having to cope alone, and simply the knowledge of having cancer.

The same patients were also asked 'What do you think has been the greatest comfort to you during your illness?' Support from family and friends was by far the commonest answer, being given by three-quarters of the patients. Other answers included medical and nursing care, religious faith, and for one woman 'Myself of course . . . I'm b-- determined.' Only two patients, both severely depressed, said everything was terrible and they had derived no comfort from anything.

## TREATMENT

When a cancer is not curable, palliative treatment with radiotherapy, chemotherapy or surgery may achieve a worthwhile relief of symptoms or prolongation of life, but these benefits need to be balanced against the side-effects and inconvenience of the treatment itself. When a patient reaches the terminal stage it is usually best to discontinue specific anticancer treatment and concentrate on relieving symptoms like pain, sleeplessness, depression or anxiety by means of appropriate drugs. Deciding when the right time to do this has arrived may be difficult, and some of the motives which guide patients to request different courses are discussed in the book by Stedeford (1984).

Determination to continue treatment right to the end may be a positive decision which reflects a 'fighting spirit' and merits respect. For other patients the same decision may be ill-founded, for example based on an extreme fear of death, or a sense of guilt about 'giving up' or letting the family down.

Similarly, a decision to stop treatment may be a reasonable one, if the patient realizes that death is inevitable and prefers to spend the end of his life quietly with the minimum of medical intervention. Other patients stop treatment from misguided motives, for example they secretly wish to die as soon as possible as a means of escape from unhappy personal circumstances which might have been improved, through counselling or social casework, if they had been revealed.

## PERSONALITY

How well a patient adjusts to having terminal cancer might be expected to depend a great deal on his personality characteristics, and how well he has coped with problems in the past. In a study of 60 married patients with terminal cancer in London (Hinton, 1975), eight aspects of previous personality were assessed through interviews with the spouses. Patients' current adjustment was gauged by their mood, attitude to illness, and satisfaction with care. Some associations between personality and current adjustment were found: patients who had previously been able to cope with problems effectively, whose marriages had been stable and happy, and who had gained satisfaction from their past life, were those best adjusted to their present illness, whereas those described as more 'neurotic' in the past were more likely to be depressed, anxious, angry or dissatisfied. However, the differences were quite small.

## RELIGION

Religious conviction, and belief in an afterlife, were found to have only weak associations with good adjustment to terminal cancer in the study by Hinton (1975) quoted above. The 50 Southampton continuing-care patients were asked whether they had a religious faith, and if so how much this had helped them cope with their illness. Their answers divided them into three groups of roughly equal size. The 18 patients in the first group had a strong faith which had been a major source of comfort to most of them:

'If it wasn't for my faith, I would have got depressed.'
'When the Lord is ready to take me, he will.'
'I know God must have had some reason for this.'

Most of this group said their faith had become stronger since they became ill and two, formerly Church of England, had changed to Roman Catholicism and Spiritualism respectively. A few expressed doubts or said their faith was weaker, and a third of this group were severely depressed despite their faith:

'I must say I do wonder how God could let me go through this.'
'I just don't know any more.'

The second group, 14 patients, had a nominal religious belief which they did not regard as an important factor in helping them adjust, and the rest had none:

'I'd like a faith, but what's the point of believing a lie?'


## DOCTOR-PATIENT COMMUNICATION

For terminal patients, communication problems 'cause more suffering than any other problem except unrelieved pain' (Stedeford, 1981b). In Stedeford's study of terminal patients in Oxford, difficulties in communication with hospital staff were more common than those involving GPs, hospice staff, or spouses. The usual complaint was being told too little or too late, but a few patients thought they had been told too much, or had been upset by learning their diagnosis in a casual manner or even accidentally. The discussion emphasizes that although many patients ask how long they have to live, it is best for doctors not to specify an exact period of time because such predictions are frequently wrong or else misinterpreted by patients, so that plans made accordingly only lead to problems.

Sixty terminal cancer patients were asked if they were satisfied with the discussion they had had with staff about their diagnosis (Hinton, 1974). Of 39 who had received complete or partial information, all were satisfied: of 21 who had been told little or nothing or given false reassurance, nine were dissatisfied. This summary of the results necessarily involves some oversimplification of the fluctuating opinions and contradictory statements which were observed in many cases.

The question 'Have the doctors told you as much as you would like to know about your illness?' was put to 43 patients in Southampton just after they had been admitted to the continuing-care unit. About half spoke openly about having incurable cancer, though few answered with such stark frankness as the man who said 'Yes, I know I'm heading for the crematorium.' Most of the rest dealt with the question indirectly: 'Yes, I suppose so . . . I can't help but be sad when I think of my son's future,' or evaded it 'Well, I've had a couple of ops, and now they're taking me down to X-ray my back.' Three wanted more information, but three thought they had been told too much: 'I wasn't ready to be told . . . I did ask but I didn't expect that answer . . . when he said cancer I just broke right down.' Two said they knew nothing and did not want to: 'I know what I want to know and that's enough.'

One study based on direct observation of doctors and nurses talking with terminally ill patients (Maguire, 1985) identified several common 'distancing tactics' which staff use to discourage patients from disclosing their psychological concerns, and so protect their own emotional equilibrium. These doctors and nurses seldom inquired directly about patients' psychological adjustment. Since few patients disclose their emotional problems spontaneously, many cases in which distress was present must have been missed. When emotional distress did come to their attention, the staff often fended off deeper discussion. Sometimes they did this by advising the patient to talk to someone else, such as the social worker, instead; sometimes they changed the subject, often diverting the conversation towards physical symptoms; in other cases they offered bland generalizations and false reassurance, or tried to 'jolly patients along'. 'Everybody feels upset when they first come in here, but you'll soon get used to it' (to a patient who had wanted to talk about her imminent death). 'You are bound to be upset with getting so much pain' (to a patient whose distress was not due to pain, but to worry about what would happen to her dog if she died). 'I'm sure we can relieve your pain' (when this was by no means certain). 'There's no need to look so glum, the sun's shining and it's a lovely day.' None of these responses enable patients' real concerns to be tackled. An even more effective 'distancing tactic', often used on general wards, is to put dying patients into side rooms and miss them out on ward rounds.

Ways to help staff deal with emotional issues more effectively are discussed in the same paper. Selection of staff is important, for those who can be flexible, are willing to share their work problems with colleagues, are realistic about the goals which can be achieved in terminal care, and whose own personal lives contain supportive relationships and varied interests, are likely to be able to do their job well without too much personal cost. In contrast, the most highly ambitious, dedicated professionals, whose approach to their work is solitary and single-minded, may not cope so well when they cannot fulfil their unrealistic ideals. Failure to cope may not be expressed directly, but shows in irritability, resentfulness, obstinacy, cynicism or black humour, minor physical symptoms and insomnia: signs of 'burn out.' Staff training can help through providing video demonstrations of interviewing and counselling skills, with opportunity for 'feedback' about students' performance. Staff at any level of experience can benefit from support groups in which problems can be discussed and shared.

## DEPRESSION

Depression in cancer patients generally has been considered in detail already (Section II.7). The frequency of depression in the 50 Southampton continuing-care patients was estimated using a short self-rating scale, the HAD, designed for physically ill patients (Zigmond and Snaith, 1983), and a brief interview. A quarter were found to be severely depressed, and two of these volunteered a request for euthanasia. Half had some depressive symptoms but were not overwhelmed by them, often commenting that they managed to fight the depression and keep cheerful. The remaining quarter claimed they were not depressed at all, making various explanatory statements:

'Plenty of others are worse off than me.'
'You've just got to accept it.'
'Nobody likes looking at a long face.'

Table 6. Factors examined in relation to depressed mood for 50 patients with terminal cancer

---

Depression more likely
  Male sex
  Older age
  In pain
  Extreme physical dependence
  Cognitive impairment
  Poorly informed about illness
  Dissatisfied with doctor-patient communication
  Recent bereavement

Depression less likely
  Past history of depression
  Living alone
  Strong religious faith
  Cerebral metastases

---

Note: all these are non-significant.

All the depressed patients attributed their depression directly to their illness, and depression had no statistically significant association with any of the other factors examined. A few trends were found (Table 6) which might have arisen due to chance in this rather small sample. The lack of any clear associations might also have arisen because some factors 'cut both ways', for example although being widowed usually increases vulnerability to depression, it might help a terminal cancer patient to face his own death more readily and therefore be less likely to become depressed.

Only a quarter of severely depressed patients in this series had had antidepressant drugs before admission to the unit, suggesting that the depression had not been recognized in the majority of cases.

## FAMILY RELATIONSHIPS

Although most terminal cancer patients regard their relatives as their chief source of support, difficulties within families are often present as well. The most common difficulties reported by the patients in our study were fear of being a burden, distress over being no longer able to care for relatives who needed them, and worry over telling relatives, especially young children, how serious the illness was.

A number of other problems were found among families in this situation referred for psychotherapy (Stedeford, 1981a&b). Anger about the illness can be inappropriately displaced towards relatives. Insecurity can lead patients to fear their partners are rejecting them in favour of someone healthy and attractive and, of course, sometimes this really does happen. Relatives may either exaggerate the patient's dependency, or go to the opposite extreme and 'deny' the illness, expecting them to carry on as before. Patients may resent watching relatives take over roles which used to be theirs, for example driving the car. The mistaken belief that cancer is 'catching' may lead either patients or relatives to shrink away from physical contact. Withdrawal from close family relationships forms a natural prelude to death for some patients, for example they find it easier to die in hospital than at home, and relatives may misinterpret this as a rejection. Some young adults 'regress' during a terminal illness and turn to their parents, which is hurtful for their spouse.

Communication between husband and wife was examined for 60 terminal cancer patients (Hinton, 1981). Only a third had spoken openly of dying to their spouse, though many others had discussed it openly with other people; another third had touched on it indirectly, using phrases which indicated ambivalence, denial and uncertainty; and a third had not discussed it with their spouse at all. The patients who did talk about dying were more certain that death was inevitable, had more 'nervous' personalities, and less good marriages. The discussion section of this paper states that it would be misleading to interpret these findings as simple 'failure of communication', for lack of discussion between patient and spouse often seemed to be a positive choice made in order to prevent distress and maintain hope, and it was not associated with any greater degree of depression or anxiety in the patients. Half the marriages in this series had grown closer since the illness.

## BEREAVED RELATIVES

After the patient with terminal cancer dies, repercussions for the relatives continue. Emotional reactions to bereavement in general usually follow a series of stages (Parkes, 1975, 1985). For the first few hours or days the bereaved person feels emotionally numb, despite an intellectual appreciation that the death has occurred. This stage is usually less marked if death was due to cancer, or other prolonged serious illness, than it is in the case of sudden unexpected deaths. When the numbness wears off, acute mental and physical distress follows: the bereaved person is tearful and restless, often feeling irrational impulses to search for the deceased or having illusions of hearing his voice or seeing his face. There may be anger towards the dead person for 'leaving', or towards the medical staff who failed to save his life. Other bereaved people feel guilt about their own failings in the relationship. A prolonged phase of depression follows the acute distress. If all goes well, the survivor becomes fully able to accept the loss, sometimes even emerging as more resourceful and resilient than before, but it may take months or years to reach this final stage.

Bereavement reactions may 'go wrong' in various ways. Some people, idealizing the memory of the dead person and not really accepting that he has died, never manage to take up an independent life of their own; others rush into a hasty remarriage or other substitute relationship without coming to terms with the loss of the first. Depressive illness, distinguishable from normal grief by its characteristic symptoms as well as by an unusually severe and prolonged depression of mood, may develop. Other illnesses, both physical and mental, are also more common in the months following bereavement. Symptoms resembling those of the deceased person's last illness may develop, and give rise to hypochondriacal fears of cancer in the survivor.

The effects of bereavement vary depending on the way in which the survivor was related to the dead person. Death of a child is usually regarded as one of the worst forms of bereavement, because parents are unprepared for having to face this reverse of the natural order, and because they often feel irrational guilt about having failed to protect someone for whose care they were responsible. I will summarize two studies about how parents respond to losing a child from cancer.

The parents of 20 children who had died from leukaemia in San Francisco were interviewed some years later (Binger *et al.,* 1969). Most of them said that learning the diagnosis had been the greatest blow, provoking depression, anger or guilt which lasted several weeks before they began to accept the situation and focus their energies into meeting all the special needs of the child. They all appreciated the fact that the hospital concerned had included them in a conference where the child's case was discussed in detail. Dissatisfactions were usually concerned with the final period of inpatient care, for example they perceived the staff as showing a formal or impatient attitude when death approached: these staff were probably trying to cope with their own distress and sense of failure by adopting a remote facade. Nearly all the parents believed the child was aware of impending death, even if this had not been discussed. When the child suspected the truth but realized the parents did not want him to know, family relationships were often strained. In two of these cases there was a big improvement after the child was told he had incurable leukaemia. Anticipation of the child's death caused the parents great distress which sometimes seemed needlessly magnified because their fantasies were more gruesome than the reality proved to be, and discussion with staff might have helped dispel these groundless fears. The death itself was not always the worst event, because so much anticipatory grieving had already been done, and because death brought an end to the child's suffering and the parents' anxiety. Some of the fathers coped with their distress by avoiding discussion of the illness and concentrating on outside activites, leaving the mothers unsupported, but three-quarters of the couples said they found support from each other. In half the families, other healthy children developed behaviour problems or psychosomatic symptoms, and also in half the families the grandparents were perceived as a hindrance rather than a support. The main recommendations these parents would make for others would be to treat the sick child 'normally', and tell the diagnosis to all the children in the family who were old enough to understand.

Twenty-four parents in Arizona who had had a child die from cancer about two years previously were sent a postal questionnaire (Shanfield *et al.,* 1984). The responses were surprisingly positive, for about half reported 'personal growth' on such measures as better ability to talk about emotional issues, more productivity and contentment, and stronger religious belief. Most families had become closer since the death, and psychiatric symptoms in the parents were hardly more common than in the general population. However, 17 parents reported continuing grief. Mothers tended to be more badly affected than fathers. Parents who had been very close to their children, though they reported more grief, had less guilt and fewer psychiatric symptoms than those who had not had such a good relationship.

# 2. Long-Term Survival

The experience of surviving cancer and being presumed cured is perceived by some patients as a positive experience which enhances their lives, by some as a disastrous trauma which they never overcome, and by others as a temporary setback with little lasting impact.

Many long-term survivors consider they have benefited from coming through the illness. Most subjects in a retrospective study of unexpectedly long survival (Kennedy *et al.*, 1976) considered themselves more appreciative of life, less concerned with trivialities, and saw the illness as 'a good experience for character development.'

The problems which other long-term survivors experience are reviewed by Naysmith *et al.*, (1983). Some of them are unable to accept their good fortune and spend the rest of their lives haunted by the spectre of malignant disease. They adopt a permanent invalid role although they have no medical reason to do so, are constantly on watch for signs and symptoms of recurrent cancer, or preoccupied with guilt and anxiety about why they should have been singled out to develop cancer in the first place. Features about cancer on TV or in magazines reinforce these preoccupations.

'Routine' follow-up in outpatient clinics can help perpetuate such patients' fears. One man wrote about his wife's reaction: 'She dreaded these visits, which subjected her to tremendous strain for the two or three weeks leading up to what proved to be an hour's wait, a short examination and a perfunctory "That's fine, see you again in six months." ' Other patients, of course, react in an opposite fashion and welcome the reassurance which continued follow-up brings.

Those who survive cancer may encounter prejudice and stigma from ill-informed acquaintances, neighbours, employers, colleagues, and insurance companies. Sometimes this is real, sometimes it mainly exists in the patient's imagination. About a quarter of the patients in my breast cancer series isolated themselves from all but very close relatives after their mastectomy, because they feared they would be rejected, but very few actual examples of rejection were given and most patients were pleasantly surprised by other people's warm acceptance when they did start mixing again. Even if deliberate stigmatization is rare, other people's ignorance can have damaging effects. Children and young adults, for example, can face extra problems following successful treatment for cancer because parents, teachers or employers fail to accept they are going to be cured. Schooling will have been interrupted for long periods during the illness, and nobody bothers to help the child catch up on education because it is assumed he will die before long. Young adults may miss chances of promotion, or lose their jobs and find it difficult to get other employment because of their medical history.

Children with leukaemia can often be cured nowadays but, paradoxically, this striking improvement in prognosis does not seem to have been accompanied by much reduction in their parents' mental distress. Instead of having to face the certainty of early death for their child, they have to cope with years of anticipating a possible relapse, which some find even more difficult.

As long-term survival becomes more common for cancer patients as a result of further advances in treatment, the psychological and social handicaps associated with having had this disease should diminish.

# 3. Can Psychological Factors Affect Cancer Prognosis?

**INTRODUCTION**

This final section contains a brief review of the evidence that psychological factors like mood, attitude, social circumstances, and life event experience can affect the course of a cancer once it has been diagnosed and treated. There is a book on this subject by Stoll (1979).

From case histories such as the two following examples from my series of patients with lung cancer, it is easy to conclude that 'lack of will to live' really does result in premature death:

*1. A retired meter reader in his early 70's had been mildly depressed, bored, and lonely since being widowed six years previously. He developed chest pains, and said that when he was told his X-ray showed a shadow 'My mind leapt to cancer.' He had the affected lung removed with the aim of cure but he died a week later. Postmortem did not explain the reason for his death, and did not detect any spread of tumour outside the lung.*
*2. A taxi driver in his late 50's had a year's history of cough and breathlessness. His wife and two brothers had all died in the year before these symptoms started. He said he 'just accepted' all the deaths. Although he had privately suspected his true diagnosis of lung cancer, he did not question the doctors about this, and was told it was 'fibrosis'. He had just finished a course of palliative radiotherapy when he coughed up a large amount of blood and died.*
Other case histories, however, show that some patients die rapidly despite a 'positive' mental attitude:

*A married administrator in his early 60's presented with one month's history of neck swelling. Otherwise he felt fit. Interviewed before bronchoscopy, he said 'Don't let's beat about the bush, this is cancer — after all, this is 1983.' He described a happy and successful past life, had no past psychiatric history, and scored zero on the depression scale. Investigations revealed lung cancer of 'oat cell' type and he began chemotherapy. In spite of intensive treatment the tumour continued to progress and he only lived three weeks.*

Physical factors like the histological type of cancer, and how advanced it was at the time of diagnosis, are known to account for much of the variation in prognosis between one patient and another. But for any individual, the growth rate of a cancer can change over time, and periods of rapid growth are sometimes interspersed with periods of 'dormancy' when little or no multiplication of cancer cells is taking place. Such fluctuations are partly dependent on the state of the tumour's environment within the body, for example the current state of the patient's immune defence system or hormone balance, factors which are partly influenced by emotional state (Editorial, 1985).

Difficulties in interpreting clinical studies on this topic arise from the impossibility of distinguishing cause and effect. For example, several of the studies described below suggest that the more passive, helpless or miserable patients have a worse prognosis, and the natural conclusion is that their spineless attitude has permitted their cancer to progress unrestrained. But it could be the other way round, and they could already have undetected tumour spread which is sapping their mental strength. Similarly, if a cancer patient deteriorates shortly after a distressing 'life event', one has to consider the possibility that this event only occurred in the first place because undetected spread of the tumour had changed the patient's behaviour, for example causing him to lose his job or contributing to the breakdown of his marriage.

Studies on this topic can be divided into two groups, the first considering factors like mood and attitude which are largely 'internal' to the patient's psychology, and the second considering more 'external' factors like social circumstances and life event stress, though the two groups clearly overlap.

## MOOD AND ATTITUDE

A retrospective study from America (Kennedy *et al.,* 1976) investigated the attitudes associated with an excellent prognosis through interviews with 22 patients who had presented 5-10 years earlier with advanced cancers, usually testicular tumours, which were expected to be rapidly fatal, but had achieved complete and lasting remissions after treatment. Most of them said that after the initial shock of their diagnosis they had conceived a powerful determination to fight their disease, and had been convinced that with the help of medical science, or of God, they were going to succeed. The other studies in this section are all prospective ones, and most have yielded rather similar findings.

A group of 204 patients with advanced cancer of the breast, cervix or lung was studied in America (Stavraky, 1968) and the longest survival times were found among those who showed 'strong hostile drives without loss of emotional control.' Another American study carried out on advanced cancer of various kinds (Weisman and Worden, 1975) showed that patients who lived longer than expected tended to have less emotional distress, closer personal relationships, and coped with their illness well, whereas the short-time survivors were distinguished by passivity and 'stoic acceptance.'

In an English study on early breast cancer (Greer *et al.,* 1979), 69 women were divided into four groups according to their expressed attitude towards their disease. Patients in two of the groups, 'fighting spirit' and 'denial', were less likely to die or develop a recurrence than patients in the other two, 'stoic acceptance' and 'helplessness/hopelessness.' As far as it was possible to tell, these attitudes were independent of the degree of advancement of the tumour at the time of initial treatment. They were, however, found to be related to patterns of immunoglobulin, which help to determine the body's resistance against cancer.

Women who already had metastases from breast cancer, and were receiving chemotherapy, were given psychological tests in an American study (Derogatis *et al.,* 1979). The 13 who lived less than a year showed less hostility, and more 'positive' emotions like joy, contentment, and affection, than the 22 long-term survivors who showed more hostility, anxiety, depression, and guilt. The long-term survivors were more likely to be judged 'poorly adjusted' by their doctors, and had less harmonious relationships with them. Though long and short survivors were similar on most physical characteristics, the short survivors in this study had had more previous chemotherapy and would have had a worse prognosis on this account alone.

Melanoma patients have been found to survive longer if they report having had to make a big emotional adjustment to cope with their illness (Rogentine *et al.,* 1979).

Many of these studies, then, have found that patients who express their emotions freely, and show an active determination to fight their disease, tend to live longer than the meek, passive, compliant or defeatist types. Some work in this field is difficult to interpret because the investigators, instead of describing the patients' mood or attitude in defined reproducible ways, use vague terms implying value-judgements. For example, 'good adjustment' from one point of view might constitute just the sort of uncomplaining, cooperative acceptance which has been linked with a poor prognosis, whereas the more challenging aggressive stance linked with a good prognosis is labelled 'bad' by the staff providing care.

The most recent American study in this field (Cassileth *et al.,* 1985b) had a different result. Seven psychosocial variables were assessed for 204 patients with incurable cancer, and for 155 patients with early breast cancer or melanoma. These variables were: social ties and marital history, job satisfaction, use of psychotropic drugs, general life evaluation/satisfaction, subjective view of adult health, hopelessness/helplessness, and amount of adjustment required to cope with the new diagnosis. These were not found to be related to survival time for the first group, and they did not help to predict the development of recurrence in the second.

## SOCIAL CIRCUMSTANCES AND LIFE EVENTS

The prognosis of 208 American women with early breast cancer was examined in relation to psychosocial measures during the five years before diagnosis (Funch and Marshall, 1983), and the results were analysed separately for three age groups. For the oldest group, death, illness or unemployment of someone in the household in this period was associated with a short survival time. This was not so for the youngest group, for whom 'subjective stress', that is feeling tired, upset, or short of money, predicted a short survival time. In the middle age group none of these measures were related to survival, perhaps because hormonal changes related to the menopause exerted such an important influence on their prognosis.

One single major life event, being widowed, was considered in a records study based on the 1971 census for England and Wales (Jones *et al.,* 1984). The sample included 108 women and 71 men who were first registered as having cancer between 1971 and 1976, and who were widowed later on in the same period. The number who died was only marginally greater than expected, the increase in mortality being larger for the widowed men than the widowed women.

## CAN CHANGING ATTITUDE IMPROVE PROGNOSIS?

If psychological factors do prove to have a role in determining cancer prognosis, there will be practical implications for patient management. The idea that it is possible to halt, or even reverse, the progression of their cancer by cultivating an active hostility towards it is inherently appealing to many patients. The appeal lies in the opportunity to gain control over the illness by individual effort. Conventional medical treatments, which merely require patients' passive cooperation, do not provide this scope for personal involvement.

Some patients spontaneously adopt measures to fight their cancer even if they know nothing about research on this topic.

Strategies which American women with breast cancer often use to give them a sense of mastery over their disease are described by Taylor (1983). Some convince themselves that their cancer was caused by eating the wrong foods or being under too much stress, and change their diet or lifestyle accordingly: if the cancer recurs despite these changes they often find a reason to disprove their original theory and become just as strongly convinced about a different one. Other patients set time aside each day to practise mental warfare against the disease: one patient continually repeated 'Body, cut this shit out.'

'Alternative therapies' for cancer are attractive because they fulfil patients' desires for more responsibility and active involvement in the management of their disease. Patients often tend to assume that treatments which demand much effort or sacrifice are the most effective. This assumption is quite illogical and some alternative treatments, for example a diet largely consisting of carrot juice, are positively harmful to health.

At present there is no convincing evidence that changing cancer patients' attitudes improves their physical prognosis, even if such changes are possible to achieve. Properly controlled studies designed to answer this question one way or the other have not yet been done. Some uncontrolled studies have claimed success, and I will summarize two of them.

A group of 225 patients with advanced cancer in America (Simonton *et al.*, 1980) received extra therapy in addition to conventional medical treatment: five-day blocks of individual and group psychotherapy every three months, and daily exercises to promote muscular relaxation, greater flexibility in thinking, release of anger and resentment, and assertive behaviour. These patients lived several months longer than expected from data on apparently similar patients treated elsewhere.

Meditation as a treatment for cancer has been advocated on the basis that profound and sustained reduction in anxiety should lead to lowered production of the hormone cortisone, which inhibits immune reactions (Meares, 1979). Patients in this study were taught meditation techniques in a small group, and advised to practise them alone for at least an hour daily. The 17 patients who participated in this programme were all reported to have survived several months longer than expected, and case histories of six whose physical symptoms improved dramatically are described.

## COMMENT

For patients who find them attractive, measures like positive thinking and meditation should probably be encouraged, so long as conventional treatment is continued at the same time. Increasing patients' sense of participation in the fight against cancer usually leads to improved psychological adjustment even if it has no direct effect on the cancer process itself.

When the psychological approach is misused, however, unhappiness or even tragedy can result. Some patients are highly vulnerable to exploitation by those alternative practitioners who, whether through their own unfounded convictions or for financial gain, encourage them to abandon conventional treatment in favour of scientifically untested but intuitively appealing measures. Other patients find any psychological approach quite alien, and are only made to feel embarrassed or inadequate if they are forced to adopt one. There is a real danger that the evidence concerning psychological influences on cancer is distorted so that, when treatment fails, both patients and their relatives are left with an unjustified extra burden of guilt.

## SUMMARY

There is some evidence that cancer patients who adopt an optimistic fighting stance against their illness have a better prognosis than those who react with passive acceptance or helpless despair. Investigations now in progress should determine whether such attitudes are truly independent rather than a reflection of already advanced disease: whether the attitudes associated with a poor prognosis can be changed and, if so, whether this leads to improved survival.

# Appendix: Breast Cancer — Patients' Own Accounts

I wrote to some of the breast cancer patients who had taken part in research interviews with me 2-5 years earlier, asking if they would care to contribute an account of their own experiences to this book. The contributions I received are reproduced here without comment or alteration by me. They cannot be fully representative, in that they come from those women who have remained in good health and who were willing to write, but they do illustrate a varied range of reactions to this common disease and its treatment.

## CASE 1 (AGE 63)

I chiefly remember how unreal it all seemed — I could hardly believe it was true and happening to me, mainly I think because there was no pain and no warning in the early stages. Later I found the pain easy to accept (compared to some others).

It was, of course, a disconcerting time, the worst perhaps waiting a week before the operation, not knowing whether it would be all taken off, or not, or only part — or what. I think I disliked the radiotherapy most of all, although I was lucky in that it did not affect me as much as some, and I was able to drive myself the odd 28 miles three days a week for the treatment. Probably I learnt to take big crises calmly as a Ferry Pilot during the War, and I am sure my mother helped when, at 16 years old she sat all night holding a deep cut on my face together, after a car accident, so that they would not put in stitches. Looking back I think I feel a deep sense of gratitude to our excellent National Health Service, and the huge amount of money spent on me at the nation's expense. The splendid hospital organization throughout and diligent after checking has been a great comfort, as one remembers every morning and night when dressing that it really *did* happen, and could happen again, and all lumps are suspicious however innocent looking. The concern of one's family and friends, especially the rather desperate anxiety and love of my only son were indeed both surprising and gratifying. It has all made me feel very deeply for those less fortunate than myself, and to realize how precious good health is to us all, though most of us take it for granted.

## CASE 2 (AGE 65 YEARS)

It was just over 5 years ago that I discovered a lump in my breast and immediately made an appointment to see my GP. Although I had no pain and felt perfectly well he arranged for an examination at the Royal South Hants Hospital. I was quite worried at first, but with reassurance and trust in all the doctors concerned, I had no hesitation in agreeing to have an operation if cancer was confirmed.

I have such praise for all the doctors and nurses during my short stay in hospital. I found it a bit of an ordeal going through the radiotherapy treatment but stuck it out and am pleased to say I had no ill-effects. My life has not changed at all since my operation as I still do a lot of gardening, painting and decorating, shopping, cooking etc.

My relations were very concerned when first hearing that I had cancer, but as I felt perfectly all right they need not have worried too much.

My advice to anyone else who has to undergo a similar operation is to keep busy and try not to think about it.

## CASE 3 (AGE 38)

I think the first reaction I had after I had been told was one of total disbelief — after all, although I had discussed the problem of breast cancer with my friends and colleagues, I didn't really think it would ever happen to me. I did ask if I could be treated in some way other than having the breast removed, but the doctor explained that if I wanted to live it was the only sure way of treating breast cancer. Well of course after that the thought of losing a breast was nothing compared to losing one's life and I just wanted to get into hospital and have the offending lump removed. After the initial shock, I felt very angry about it — how dare it invade my body, I even asked the surgeon what had happened to it because I felt like I wanted to destroy it like it had nearly destroyed me! Then of course I questioned everything that I had done in the previous months. Was it because I had gone jogging! — or was it because I had plucked a long hair that had grown by my nipple! Lots of silly things went through my mind.

The staff at the hospital were fantastic, so kind and cheerful — I really felt I was in to have my tonsils out as no big fuss was made, and this made me realize that it wasn't the end of the world, that lots of women had this done every week and survived. Sister X who looks after all the ladies who have the mastectomy operation was super, there wasn't one question unanswered and not one I felt I could not ask her. I can't speak too highly of her, I don't think that I could have coped without her. She encouraged my husband to talk about it and made me realize that it is just as traumatic for the man as well as for the woman. We discussed how I would cope with making love afterwards, would I feel the same as before? as I'm sure most women would imagine that they would feel less than a perfect person after, and although it is a shock to see yourself afterwards it didn't make any difference to my husband at all — he still thinks I'm sexy!

With regards to the operation itself, I was most surprised to find that it affected my arm, I wasn't expecting that part of my body to hurt. I have since had the breast reconstruction operation. It was a great success and I'm really pleased with it. It's only after you get the new breast do you realize how much you missed the other one!

It's two years now since it happened, and unfortunately I have a lump in my other breast. I am waiting for an appointment at the hospital, and I am keeping my fingers crossed that it will turn out to be something simple. But if it's not then at least I shall be prepared this time, and I know I can survive.

## CASE 4 (AGE 47)

It is five and a half years since breast cancer was diagnosed and I was operated on, now I am fit and well and go for a check up once a year. Like most women I just could not believe it when breast cancer was diagnosed — you think it can only happen to other people. But after the initial shock things moved so quickly there was not a lot of time to worry. Everyone I came in contact with was so kind and helpful, especially the nurses. The other things which mean so much to a woman in this position is having a loving, caring husband and the back up of a supportive family and friends.

I have been able to help friends and relations facing the same problem by just being someone who has had the experience and can offer a sympathetic ear and answer a few questions. A sister-in-law has recently had the operation and I was able to give her confidence, also more recently my own daughter who is 27 had a small lump removed which proved to be cancerous. She has had the option of keeping her breast or plastic surgery, which I very much would like to have had.

The other thing I must mention is the after care department; this is another helpful part of the hospital and gets top marks from me.

I am now enjoying life to the full, grandchildren to babysit for and various spare time activities, also as my husband is retired we have our fair share of holidays.

## CASE 5 (AGE 40)

At first when I was told that I had cancer of the breast my first reaction was that under no circumstances would I have it off.

After I had discussed it with my husband and family doctor I realized that I had to go ahead and have the op.

My first thoughts and fears were that it would change my husband's feelings for me but he did say it would not make any difference to him or the way he felt about me — I don't think that I could have accepted the fact that I had lost a breast if it had not been for the help and support of my husband and family at this time.

I did find that the doctors and nurses were very good and that the follow-up in the outpatients dept was different than any other dept that I have visited before or since. The atmosphere is so friendly and the staff seem to make you feel as if you are the only one in this position even though there are so many other people there. I'm sure that this helped me a lot. My friends wanted to know about the op and were very interested to see what the scar was like; I think it is a help if you can talk about it instead of hiding away and feeling sorry for yourself.

I do think that there should be more information that should be given out at school to get the girls of the next generation to check their breasts earlier.

## CASE 6 (AGE 60)

I was aware of the breast cancer statistics and having convinced myself my little lump was just a cyst, it was a great shock to learn that the breast would have to be removed. I was grateful there was someone available to help me make the hospital admission arrangements.

I cried a lot and prayed a lot. My husband and I talked a lot, about our feelings, our love and concern for each other. I concluded I could cope with this problem despite disfigurement, which even at 60 years of age was important to me. But I was very worried about any further problems. I tried to concentrate on leaving everything in good order, including my will and being an only child, instructions regarding my aged mother's affairs.

I was apprehensive about the operation, but had confidence in the surgeon's skill and the nursing care. Normally of a cheerful disposition, the tears were never far away, but helped by the companionship of the other patients.

My two daughters were very concerned and were as supportive as possible considering the considerable distances between us, and with young families. I shall always be grateful to the Breast Care Sister who was a sympathetic listener and adviser and felt her telephone number could be a lifeline. I was not enthusiastic about going to the convalescent home, but the two weeks I spent there were very beneficial, both physically and mentally.

I was lucky, a successful operation and no further treatment, but still felt I would never lead a life free from anxiety, but have tried to live, as advised, one day at a time, and gradually my fears have receded. The periodic checkups are reassuring. Relatives and friends were kind, which was appreciated, but I was so fortunate in having the practical and moral support of a caring husband.

## CASE 7 (AGE 48)

What a shock it was to learn that just one month before our planned holiday abroad I would have to go into hospital to have this 'lump' removed, which both my GP and the hospital consultant thought was just a reoccurrence of mastitis. Apparently the mammogram had shown it was not as innocent as was at first thought and in my ignorance I was not aware that the mammogram showed anything than just a 'lump'. I wasn't told on my recall to the hospital that it would almost certainly be a mastectomy but could tell from the Doctor's attitude that it would be. I explained that my holiday was imminent and that I would like to go and then have the operation when I returned. He said no and so it was arranged for me to go in the following week to have the operation on the Tuesday.

I naturally spent a very apprehensive week waiting for the 'big day' and I must say I was more concerned about my family, knowing how worried they all were, so I just carried on as normal, going to work and doing all the usual things. Everybody was so helpful and kind, those people who knew! As I explained, it wasn't going to be a secret but on the other hand I wasn't going to shout it from the rooftops.

After the operation the one big question was, was it the big 'op' and yes it was, but due to all the help and kindness shown in the hospital I was able to go home on the Friday. I had lots of visitors that weekend, some planned and others casual who didn't know I had been in hospital. This was all very tiring and I wouldn't recommend too many visitors, as they are not aware of how tired one feels. In the weeks to follow I was sore and uncomfortable and my arm was so stiff I couldn't wash properly, a very common complaint I understand. I had to go for a bone scan one week after the operation, nothing painful but quite tiring. From then on I made good enough progress to be able to go on that holiday and although the journey was tiring, the two weeks in the sun and plenty of gentle swimming did me the world of good, so much so that I was able to go back to work just six weeks after the operation.

At the beginning I did feel that it was a question of living life to the full 'just in case' but now feel, nearly six years on, that I can plan for the future. I was so lucky that the cancer was caught early and that I had no need for any follow-up treatment, and I am now on annual visits only.

## CASE 8 (AGE 46)

When I was told I had breast cancer I felt cold with fear. I just did not want to believe it, it was as if the specialist was talking to someone else not me, although he was very kind. Thoughts came rushing into my head of not seeing my children married or seeing my grandchildren come along. My husband and I clung to each other when we got home and cried, afterwards we talked and talked each afraid not for ourselves but for the other one. My husband's fear was of losing me and that he felt helpless, wanting to say something to make me less afraid and knowing he couldn't.

The operation itself was no problem. I felt a bit weak but was never allowed to be in any pain as pain killers were always available. When the bandages first came off I was very reluctant to look and when I did my unreal feelings returned, however as the days passed I began to think how lucky I was to be alive and my natural determination returned, I was dreading my husband seeing me for the first time but I was in a nursing home for two weeks and a very kind nurse suggested perhaps my husband might like to sit in with me when my dressing was changed. This helped a lot as having seen the scar at its worst I knew that every time from then on it could only look better. When I came home I was bright as could be for the first week, then came two weeks when I did nothing but cry. I have the kindest, gentlest of husbands but nothing he did was right; either I said he fussed too much or he didn't fuss enough. I must have been awful to live with but just couldn't stop. After two weeks of crying and sleeping the old me returned and I never looked back. Now two years after my operation I can't think of anything I used to do that I can't do again now. I still confess to feeling a little sadness when I see myself naked at bathtime, but there is more to life than a beautiful body — cancer taught me that.

## CASE 9 (AGE 51)

Looking back, when I first discovered something was wrong I could not bring myself to confide in anyone, not even my husband. I kept it to myself for several weeks, hoping I was imagining it. I had no pain, the first sign was my nipple being drawn inwards.

It was while taking my grandson to see the doctor, I decided to ask the nurse on duty to examine my breasts. The nurse immediately called in a doctor, and within three days I had an appointment to see Professor X at his clinic. Within two weeks I was in hospital to have as I thought a biopsy, being told vaguely, that there was no cause for concern. It was therefore rather a shock after coming from the operating theatre, to be told it was necessary for me to have had a mastectomy, although in my sub-conscious I rather expected just that.

The attention I received from the hospital staff, and the staff at the clinic, was excellent; had I been a private patient I could not have received better treatment. The understanding of my family helped me tremendously, it has made no difference to my marriage at all.

## CASE 10 (AGE 48)

Re my feelings 2 years ago:
1. Shock — disbelief that it could or should happen to me.
2. Acceptance of a situation to be talked over and discussed by my husband, family, friends, and colleagues.
3. I think it helped me that I am a Community Sister and knew about the course and procedure of hospitals, wards, tests, examinations, etc. which had to be performed before and after. Knowing (or hoping I knew) it wise to have a complete removal of breast plus glands of axilla to give the surgeon a chance to remove the malignancy and be able to assess the extent of malignancy. I had seen patients who had received perhaps lumpectomy, radiotherapy, etc. without success and my one thought was to rid myself of the offending part of my body and the chance to live a longer life (hopefully) through the operation.

I could not have had a better selection of doctors, nurses, even cleaners and fellow patients to go through the experience with. Unfortunately I picked up an infection 1 week after the operation treated quickly by antibiotics but instead of a flat scar, I have a 'pucker' at one end. I do experience tightening of my left side breast area and upper arm every time my menstrual period is due — otherwise with a super prothesis I have maintained my confidence, etc. and can now talk to some patients who are experiencing worries, etc. in our day surgery where I work.

I received a visit from a fellow community sister while I was waiting for my operation for which I was grateful. She had had a mastectomy and reconstruction 10 years ago successfully. I will not be having a reconstruction but I can understand why some women feel they would like to try — younger than myself perhaps with grand-children — sporty type wearing swimsuits etc.

The leaflets I received at the time were helpful — not only to myself but more to my husband and family to try to understand. I think well women/men clinics should be more available and hopefully will be in the future. We have a very good clinic which I attended every 2-4 months and now 6 monthly.

## CASE 11 (AGE 48)

From the time my general practitioner received the adverse mammogram result, through the hurriedly arranged appointment at the breast clinic, to the day of the frozen section and subsequent operation with its inevitable result I think my nurse's training helped me to accept more quickly and with reasonable outward calm that I had to have a mastectomy.

However, nothing in my training prepared me for the feelings which resulted from the questionnaire I was asked to complete three days before the operation when I was sent to the ward for blood tests and admission examination. This questionnaire required me to put on paper answers to questions which my state of thought and feeling did not want to acknowledge and from that time until admission I was mentally distressed and depressed. I also felt anger when I discovered the seventy-year-old lady in the next bed, who had no medical knowledge of what was happening to her, had been reduced to tears after answering the questions.

On the same day that I had my operation a friend with two teenage daughters died from breast cancer. When I read the notice in the paper the next evening it was the first time I was able to cry for her and for myself and I remember praying that I should live to see my elder daughter through college and my younger daughter reach her eighteenth birthday.

The physical problems of overcoming the operation soon became a challenge with great encouragement from all my colleagues, friends, and the community physiotherapist. The mental setback of having to accept the need for adjuvant chemotherapy was after agreement with my husband, a course that had to be taken and if it failed the need for people to take part in trials was still essential. The saying that you get used to treatment just does not apply to chemotherapy and nothing will ever make me forget the unavoidable nausea that assailed me after I arrived home on a Wednesday and lasted until Friday evening. However I was lucky enough to work in an accommodating hospital and by Saturday evening I knew I would be back on duty.

Two subsequent question and answer sessions about my feelings following the operation were accepted by me with much more equanimity than the first.

Regular follow-up appointments were at first a major hurdle, causing tension for up to a week before the visit. After five and a half years it is only as I walk through the door and am shown into one of the claustrophobic little rooms, where my memory of the intravenous injections is still as clear as ever, that I shiver. Then into the room comes Dr X with his air of nonchalant reassurance and so far all has been well again.

I must mention my high regard for the Sister who was appointed at the time I had my operation and who has been so much help to so many since that time. With her prompting I set up a local mastectomy group of about ten people. We met with great enthusiasm at first but the group was disbanded after about a year because I could see that such a peer group was bound to become too introspective. Sadly three of this group have died but four of the group went on to become committee members of a newly formed Combat Cancer group for the Wessex Cancer Trust where I thought we could all be much more positive in our outlook.

After three years I had a breast reconstruction and although I have not yet progressed to having the nipple and areola attached, the psychological benefit of having natural cleavage again is wonderful.

For a long time after the initial operation I was unable to look or plan very far ahead but I am so far, one of the lucky ones, with no adverse reactions from the chemotherapy. My present position as a practice nurse means that I am able to offer advice on the need for regular breast examination and reassurance and the benefit of experience to patients who have recently had a mastectomy, or who are faced with the possibility. My elder daughter takes her degree this year and my younger daughter will be eighteen years old in May.

If I had had no medical knowledge I could only have said that I was very grateful to all the medical and nursing staff with whom I came in contact. As a nurse I have also been grateful to have been treated by the doctors and the majority of the nurses as an equal. However I do feel that some nurses still do not appreciate the mental trauma of such an operation in their eagerness to help the patient overcome the physical disfiguration.

## CASE 12 (AGE 48)

To be told that the lump on my breast could be nasty was a dreadful shock, as like everyone else one thinks it will never happen to them. At first I felt cancer was a monster for which there was no control but at the same time I was determined to beat it.

As a family we are very close and it was then I was grateful for that. With the love and support from my husband and children I was able to make it just another challenge. It helped that the operation proved not to be nearly as bad as I imagined. I suffered no pain and healed quickly. I can remember after having my breast removed my first reaction was not to look down at the wound. I was afraid to but I had to realize there was no going back.

The doctors and nurses in particular have always been very kind and helpful at all times and even now when I go for my yearly check up one notices that the staff can't do enough to help every individual patient.

It is now five years since I had my mastectomy and I am a very fit and healthy person. For that I am grateful.

# Glossary of Medical Terms Used in Text

**Adenocarcinoma** a carcinoma originating from glandular tissue. Includes most cancers of the breast, bowel, some lung cancers, and cancers of many other organs.

**Adjuvant treatment** additional treatment, by radiotherapy or chemotherapy, given to destroy any residual cancer cells left behind after surgery.

**Affective disorders** a group of psychiatric illnesses characterized by disturbed mood, and including depressive illness and mania.

**Amitriptyline** an antidepressant drug of the 'tricyclic' group.

**Anaplastic carcinoma** a histological type of cancer, usually fast-growing.

**Androgen** male sex hormone.

**Axillary lymph nodes** the lymph nodes in the armpit, which are usually the first site for secondary deposits in breast cancer.

**Benign** non-malignant, non-cancerous.

**Biopsy** removal of a small piece of tissue for histological examination.

**Bone scan** a special X-ray to detect the presence of secondary deposits (metastases) of cancer in bones.

**Bronchitis** inflammation of the bronchi. Chronic bronchitis, usually occurring in heavy smokers, causes cough and breathlessness.

**Bronchoscopy** examination of the bronchi (air passages) in the lungs, through a tube passed down the throat.

**Carcinogenic** capable of causing cancer, or contributing to its cause.

**Carcinoma** a common type of cancer which arises from epithelial tissue.

**Cell** the smallest unit in the body which is able to function independently. Visible under a microscope.

**Cerebral** relating to the brain.

**Cervix** (adj. cervical) neck of the womb.

**Chemotherapy** drug treatment: for cancer patients, usually means cytotoxic drug treatment.

**Clinical depression** pathological depression of mood requiring treatment: depressive illness.

**Cognitive** concerned with intellectual functions such as perception, thought, memory, reasoning.

**Cognitive therapy** a form of treatment which uses reasoning processes to treat depression or anxiety.

**Colostomy** surgical formation of an opening from the colon (large bowel) onto the surface of the body. Sometimes necessary after operations to treat cancer of the colon or rectum.

**Continuing-care unit** a hospital unit for managing patients with advanced cancer.

**Cortisone** a steroid hormone produced in the adrenal gland.

**Counselling** listening to problems and offering information and advice.

**Delusion** a false belief, which is not in keeping with the beliefs of the subject's social group, and which persists irrespective of evidence against it. May occur in schizophrenia, paranoid psychoses, severe depressive illness, mania or organic brain syndromes.

**Denial** an unconscious 'mental mechanism' which involves ignoring some threatening aspect of external reality.

**ECT** electroconvulsive therapy: used to treat severe depression.

**Ego** the conscious part of the mind which deals with everyday reality (a theoretical concept associated with Sigmund Freud).

**Endogenous depression** depression which cannot be explained by stressful life circumstances.

**Euphoria** exaggerated elation.

**Genetic** inherited.

**Hallucination** a false perception arising in the absence of an appropriate external stimulus. Auditory hallucinations ('hearing voices') are characteristic of schizophrenia, paranoid psychoses, severe depressive illness, or mania. Visual hallucinations ('seeing things') are characteristic of organic brain syndromes.

**Histology** study of tissue under a microscope. Usually necessary to confirm a diagnosis of cancer.

**Hodgkin's disease** a type of lymphoma.

**Hormone** a chemical, produced by one of the endocrine glands, which circulates in the blood and exerts effects on other parts of the body.

**Hypercalcaemia** raised level of calcium in the blood. May occur as a complication of cancer.

**Hypochondriasis** excessive concern about physical health.

**Hysterectomy** removal of the womb.

Immune system the body's defence system (including lymphocytes and antibodies) against disease.

**Intellectualization** explaining emotional issues in logical, rational terms.

**Larynx** voice box.

**Latent period** the time during which a cancer is developing in the body but has not yet given rise to any signs or symptoms.

**Leukaemia** a type of cancer in which there are too many white cells in the blood, due to overactivity of bone marrow.

**Lumpectomy** removal of a cancer without removing the whole organ in which it has arisen. A term specially used for breast cancer.

**Lymph nodes** bean-shaped masses of tissue, in various parts of the body, containing *'lymphocytes'*, cells which protect against infection and other disease.

**Lymphoma** a tumour originating in lymph nodes or lymphoid tissue.

**Mania** a psychiatric illness characterized by elation of mood and overactivity.

**Mastectomy** surgical removal of a breast. Sometimes the axillary lymph nodes are removed at the same time.

**Melanoma** a form of skin cancer which develops from a mole.

**Metabolic disturbance** disturbance of body chemistry.

**Metastases** secondary deposits of cancer in parts of the body other than the organ of origin.

**Mianserin** a modern antidepressant drug.

**Mood disorders (affective disorders)** depression, anxiety or elated mood states which are inappropriate or out of proportion to circumstances.

**Neoplasm** 'new growth': often used as another word for cancer.

**Neuromyopathy** disturbed function of nerves and muscles, causing such symptoms as weakness or pain.

**Organic brain syndromes** conditions caused by physical disease of the brain itself, or by chemical disturbances (resulting from disease of other organs, or from drugs) which disturb brain function. Organic brain syndromes may cause cognitive disturbance such as impaired memory or confusion, hallucinations, delusions, and mood disturbance.

**Palliative treatment** treatment designed to bring temporary relief of symptoms when cure is not possible.

**Pancreas** an abdominal organ which produces insulin and certain enzymes required for digestion of food.

**Paranoid** suspicious, fearful of persecution.

**Paraplegia** paralysis of the lower part of the body.

**Personality** behavioural and mental traits characteristic of an individual.

**Prednisolone** a steroid drug, similar to the natural hormone cortisone, sometimes used in treatment of cancer.

**Primary site** the place in the body where a cancer originally developed.

**Projection** attributing one's own, usually unacceptable, feelings to other people.

**Prospective study** a research design in which subjects are followed up to observe relationships between their original characteristics and what happens to them later (cf. retrospective).

**Prosthesis** an artificial substitute for a missing body part.

**Psychosomatic** a description of physical symptoms which are believed to have been caused, or partly caused, by psychological factors.

**Psychotherapy** treatment through the exchange of words and feelings within a professional relationship.

**Radical treatment** intensive treatment, aimed to cure.

**Radiotherapy** treatment, usually for cancer, by high energy irradiation.

**Rationalization** an unconscious 'mental mechanism' which involves finding a logical reason for thoughts or beliefs which are really determined by emotions of an unacknowledged or unacceptable kind.

**Regression** literally 'moving backwards'. Used:

1. in cancer medicine to mean the shrinking of a tumour, for example after successful radiotherapy or chemotherapy;
2. in psychiatry to mean reverting back to feelings or behaviour appropriate to an earlier stage of life.

**Repression** an unconscious 'mental mechanism' in which some threatening or unacceptable feeling, which has briefly 'registered', becomes ignored or forgotten.

**Retrospective study** a research design in which subjects who already have the condition under study are questioned about their past, to seek possible causes (cf. prospective).

**Sarcoma** a rare type of cancer arising from connective tissue or its derivatives.

**Schizophrenia** a psychiatric illness characterized by delusions, hallucinations, withdrawal from reality, and deterioration of the personality.

**Somatic** bodily, physical.

**Squamous cell carcinoma** a cancer originating from a type of epithelial cell. Includes some cancers of the skin and lung.

**Steroid** a group of substances, including hormones from the adrenal gland and artificial chemicals, with widespread physiological effects, sometimes used in treating cancer.

**Suppression** deliberately excluding something unpleasant from one's thoughts.

**Systemic** affecting the body as a whole.

**Tamoxifen** a drug with anti-oestrogen effects, used to treat breast cancer.

**Tissue** part of the body consisting of a large number of cells having a similar structure and function.

**Tumour** an abnormal mass of tissue caused by excess growth of cells. May be cancerous (malignant) or benign (non-malignant).

# References

Abse, DW, Wilkins, MM, Van de Castle, RL, Buxton, WD, Demars, JP, Brown, RS and Kirschner, LG (1974). Personality and behavioural characteristics of lung cancer patients. *J Psychosom Res,* **18,** 101-113.

Aitken-Swan, J, and Easson, EC (1959). Reactions of cancer patients on being told their diagnosis. *Br Med J,* **i,** 779-783.

Aitken-Swan, J, and Paterson, R (1955). The cancer patient: delay in seeking advice. *Br Med J,* **i,** 623-627.

American Psychiatric Association (1980). *Diagnostic and Statistical Manual of Mental Disorders.* 3rd ed. American Psychiatric Association: Washington DC.

Barton, TT, (1965). Life after laryngectomy. *Laryngoscope,* **75,** 1408-1415.

Binger, CM, Abkin, AR, Feuerstein, RC, Kushner, JH, Zoger, S and Mikkelson, C (1969). Childhood leukaemia: emotional impact on patient and family. *N Engl J Med,* **280,** 414-418.

Box, V, Nichols, S, Lallemand, RC, Pearson, P and Vakil, PA (1984). Haemoccult compliance rates and reasons for non-compliance. *Public Health,* **98,** 16-25.

Brown, D and Pedder, J (1979). *An Introduction to Psychotherapy.* Tavistock: London.

Brown, G and Harris, T (1978). *Social Origins of Depression.* Tavistock: London.

Bukberg, J, Penman, D and Holland, JC (1984). Depression in hospitalised cancer patients. *Psychosom Med,* **46,** 199-212.

Cairns, J (1985). The treatment of diseases and the war against cancer. *Sci Am,* **253,** 5, 31-39.

Cassileth, BR, Lusk, EJ, Strouse, TB, Miller, DS, Brown, LL and Cross, PA (1985a). A psychological analysis of cancer patients and their next-of-kin. *Cancer,* **55,** 72-76.

Cassileth, BR, Lusk, EJ, Miller, DS, Brown, LL and Miller, C (1985b). Psychosocial correlates of survival in advanced malignant disease? *N Engl J Med,* **312,** 1551-1555.

Chessells, JM (1985). Cranial irradiation in childhood lymphoblastic leukaemia: time for reappraisal? *Br Med J,* **ii,** 686-687.

Craig, TJ and Abeloff, MD (1974). Psychiatric symptomatology among hospitalised cancer patients. *Am J Psychiatry,* **131**, 1323-1327.

rammer, J, Barraclough, BM and Heine, B (1982). *The Use of Drugs in Psychiatry.* Gaskell: London.

Dahlstrom, WG, Welsh, GS and Dahlstrom, LE (1975). *An MMPI Handbook.* University of Minnesota: Minneapolis.

Dattore, PJ, Shontz, FC and Coyne, L (1980). Premorbid personality differentiation of cancer and non-cancer groups: a test of the hypothesis of cancer proneness. *J Consult Clin Psychol,* **48**, 388-394.

Dean, C, Chetty, U and Forrest, AP (1983). Effects of immediate breast reconstruction on psychosocial morbidity after mastectomy. *Lancet,* **i**, 307-312.

Derogatis, LR, Abeloff, MD and Melisaratos, N (1979). Psychological coping mechanisms and survival time in metastatic breast cancer. *JAMA,* **242**, 1505-1508.

Derogatis, LR, Morrow, GR, Fetting, J, Penman, D, Piasetsky, S, Schmale, AM, Henrichs, M and Carnicke, CLM (1983). The prevalence of psychiatric disorders among cancer patients. *JAMA,* **249**, 751-757.

Devlin, HB, Plant, JA and Griffin, M (1971). Aftermath of surgery for anorectal cancer. *Br Med J,* **ii**, 413-418.

Editorial (1979). The mind and cancer. *Lancet,* **i**, 706-707.

Editorial (1985). Emotion and immunity. *Lancet,* **ii**, 133-134.

Evans, NJR, Baldwin, JA and Gath, D (1974). The incidence of cancer among patients with affective disorders. *Br J Psychiatry,* **124**, 518-525.

Forester, BM, Kornfield, DS and Fleiss, J (1978). Psychiatric aspects of radiotherapy. *Am J Psychiatry,* **135**, 960-963.

Fox, BH, Stanek, EJ, Boyd, SC and Flanney, JT (1982). Suicide rates among cancer patients in Connecticut. *J Chronic Dis,* **35**, 89-100.

Frank, JW and Mai, V (1985). Breast self-examination in young women: more harm than good? *Lancet,* **ii**, 654-657.

Fras, I, Litin, EM and Pearson, JS (1967). Comparison of psychiatric symptoms in carcinoma of the pancreas with those in some other intra-abdominal neoplasms. *Am J Psychiatry,* **123**, 1553-1562.

Funch, DP and Marshall, J (1983). The role of stress, social support and age in survival from breast cancer. *J Psychosom Res,* **27**, 77-83.

Goldberg, RJ (1981). Management of depression in the patient with advanced cancer. *JAMA,* **246**, 373-376.

Gordon, WA, Freidenbergs, I, Diller, L, Hibbard, M, Wolf, C, Levine, L, Lipkins, R, Ezrachi, O and Lucido, D. (1980). Efficacy of psychosocial intervention with cancer patients. *J Consult Clin Psychol,* **48**, 743-759.

Greer, S and Morris, T (1975). Psychological attributes of women who develop breast cancer: a controlled study. *J Psychosom Res,* **19**, 147-153.

Greer, S, Morris, T and Pettingale, KW (1979). Psychological response to breast cancer: effect on outcome. *Lancet,* **ii**, 785-787.

Hinton, J (1972). Psychiatric consultation in fatal illness. *Proc R Soc Med,* **65**, 29-32.

Hinton, J (1974). Talking to people about to die. *Br Med J,* **ii**, 25-27.

Hinton, J (1975). Influence of previous personality on reactions to having terminal cancer. *Omega,* **6**, 95-111.

Hinton, J (1981). Sharing or withholding awareness of dying between husband and wife. *J Psychosom Res,* **25**, 337-343.

Horne, RL and Picard, RS (1979). Psychosocial risk factors for lung cancer. *Psychosom Med,* **41**, 503-513.

Hughes, JE (1982). Emotional reactions to the diagnosis and treatment of early breast cancer. *J Psychosom Res,* **26**, 277-283.

Hughes, JE (1985a). Depressive illness and lung cancer. I. Depression before diagnosis. *Eur J Surg Onc,* **11**, 15-20.

Hughes, JE (1985b). Depressive illness and lung cancer. II. Follow-up of inoperable patients. *Eur J Surg Onc,* **11**, 21-24.

Hughes, JE and Lee, D (1987). Depressive symptoms in patients with terminal cancer. In: *Psychosocial Issues in Malignant Disease,* M Watson and S Greer (Eds). Pergamon Press: Oxford.

Jacobs, TJ and Charles, E (1980). Life events and the occurrence of cancer in children. *Psychosom Med,* **42**, 11-24.

Jones, DR, Goldblatt, PO and Leon, DA (1984). Bereavement and cancer: some results using data on deaths of spouses from the OPCS longitudinal study. *Br Med J,* **ii**, 461-464.

Jones, SJ (1981). Telling the right patient. *Br Med J,* **ii**, 291-293.

Kendell, RE (1981). Present status of electro convulsive therapy. *Br J Psychiatry,* **139**, 265-283.

Kennedy, J, Tellegen, A, Kennedy, S and Havernick, N (1976). Psychological response of patients cured of advanced cancer. *Cancer,* **38**, 2184-2191.

Kerr, TA, Shapira, K and Roth, M (1969). The relationship between premature death and affective disorders. *Br J Psychiatry,* **115**, 1277-1282.

Kissen, DM (1963). Personality characteristics in males conducive to lung cancer. *Br J Med Psychol,* **36**, 27-36.

Leathar, DS and Roberts, MM (1985). Older women's attitudes towards breast disease, self examination and screening facilities: implications for communication. *Br Med J,* **i**, 668-670.

Le Shan, L (1966). An emotional life-history pattern associated with neoplastic disease. *Ann NY Acad Sci,* **125**, 780-793.

Levine, PM, Silberfarb, PM and Lipowski, ZJ (1978). Mental disorders in cancer patients. *Cancer,* **42**, 1385-1391.

Lloyd, GG (1977). Psychological reactions to physical illness. *Br J Hosp Med,* **18**, 352-358.

Lloyd, GG, Parker, AC, Ludlam, CA and McGuire, RJ (1984). Emotional impact of diagnosis and early treatment of lymphomas. *J Psychosom Res,* **28**, 157-162.

Mackay, D (1982). Cognitive behaviour therapy. *Br J Hosp Med,* **27**, 242-247.

Magarey, CJ, Todd, PB and Blizard, PJ (1977). Psychosocial factors influencing delay and breast self-examination in women with symptoms of breast cancer. *Soc Sci Med,* **11**, 229-232.

Maguire, P (1984). Can the parental psychological morbidity associated with childhood leukaemia be reduced? *Cancer Surveys,* **3**, 617-631.

Maguire, P (1985). Barriers to psychological care of the dying. *Br Med J,* **ii**, 1711-1713.

Maguire, GP, Lee, EG, Bevington, DJ, Kuchemann, CS, Crabtree, RJ and Cornell, CE (1978). Psychiatric problems in the first year after mastectomy. *Br Med J,* **i**, 963-965.

Maguire, GP, Tait, A, Brooke, M, Thomas, C, Howat, JMT, Sellwood, RA and Bush, H (1980). Psychiatric morbidity and physical toxicity associated with adjuvant chemotherapy after mastectomy. *Br Med J,* **ii**, 1179-1180.

Malan, DH (1979). *Individual Psychotherapy and the Science of Psychodynamics.* Butterworth: London.

Meares, A (1979). Meditation: a psychological approach to cancer treatment. *Practitioner,* **222**, 119-122.

Meyerowitz, BE, Sparks, FC and Spears, IK (1979). Adjuvant chemotherapy for breast carcinoma: psychosocial implications. *Cancer,* **43**, 1613-1618.

Morris, T, Greer, S and White, P (1977). Psychological and social adjustment to mastectomy: a 2 year follow-up study. *Cancer,* **40**, 2381-2387.

Morris, T, Greer, S, Pettingale, KW and Watson, M (1981). Patterns of expression of anger and their psychological correlates in women with breast cancer. *J Psychosom Res,* **25**, 111-117.

Muslin, HL, Gyarfas, K and Pieper, WJ (1966). Separation experience and cancer of the breast. *Ann NY Acad Sci,* **125**, 802-806.

Naysmith, A, Hinton, JM, Meredith, R, Marks, MD and Berry, RJ (1983). Psychological and family aspects of surviving malignant disease. *Br J Hosp Med,* **30**, 22-27.

Nerenz, DR, Leventhal, H and Love, RR (1982). Factors contributing to emotional distress during cancer chemotherapy. *Cancer,* **50**, 1020-1027.

Nichols, S, Waters, WE, Fraser, JD, Wheeler, MJ and Ingham, SK (1981). Delay in the presentation of breast symptoms for consultant investigation. *Community Med,* **3**, 217-225.

Parkes, CM (1975). *Bereavement: Studies of Grief in Adult Life*. Penguin: Harmondsworth.

Parkes, CM (1985). Bereavement. *Br J Psychiatry,* **146**, 11-17.

Paykel, ES and Rao, BM (1984). Methodology in Studies of Life Events and Cancer. In *Psychosocial Stress and Cancer,* CL Cooper (Ed.). Wiley: Chichester.

Peck, A (1972). Emotional reactions to having cancer. *Am J Roentgenol Radium Ther Nucl Med,* **114**, 591-599.

Peck, A and Boland, J (1977). Emotional reactions to radiation treatment. *Cancer,* **40**, 180-184.

Peck, B (1979). Effects of childhood cancer on longterm survivors and their families. *Br Med J,* **i**, 1327-1329.

Plumb, MM and Holland, J (1977). Comparative studies of psychological function in patients with advanced cancer — I Self reported depressive symptoms. *Psychosom Med,* **39**, 264-276.

Priestman, TJ, Priestman, SG and Bradshaw, C (1985). Stress and breast cancer. *Br J Cancer,* **51**, 493-498.

Rogentine, GN, Vankammen DP, Fox, BH, Docherty, JP, Rosenblatt, JE, Boyd, SC and Bunney, WE (1979). Psychological factors in the prognosis of malignant melanoma: a prospective study. *Psychosom Med,* **41**, 647-655.

Schmale, AHJ and Iker, HP (1966). The affect of hopelessness and the development of cancer. *Psychosom Med,* **28**, 714-721.

Schonfield, J (1975). Psychological and life-experience differences between Israeli women with benign and cancerous breast lesions. *J Psychosom Res,* **19**, 229-234.

Seibel, MM, Freeman, MG and Graves, WL (1980). Carcinoma of the cervix and sexual function. *Obstet Gynecol,* **55**, 484-487.

Shanfield, SB, Benjamin, AH and Swain, BJ (1984). Parents' reactions to the death of an adult child from cancer. *Am J Psychiatry,* **141**, 1092-1094.

Shekelle, RB, Raynor, WJ, Ostfeld, MD, Garron, DC, Bieliauskas, LA, Liu, SC, Maliza, C and Paul, O (1981). Psychological depression and 17 year risk of death from cancer. *Psychosom Med,* **43**, 117-125.

Silberfarb, PM, Philibert, D and Levine, PM (1980). Psychosocial aspects of neoplastic disease. II. Affective and cognitive effects of chemotherapy in cancer patients. *Am J Psychiatry,* **137**, 597-601.

Simonton, OC, Simonton, SM and Sparks, TF (1980). Psychological intervention in the treatment of cancer. *Psychosomatics,* **21**, 226-233.

Smith, CK, Harrison, SD, Ashworth, C, Montano, D, Davis, A and Fefer, A (1984). Life change and onset of cancer in identical twins. *J Psychosom Res,* **28**, 525-532.

Smith, WR and Sebastian, H (1976). Emotional history and pathogenesis of cancer. *J Clin Psychol,* **32**, 863-866.

Spiegel, D, Bloom, JR and Yalom, I (1981). Group support for patients with metastatic cancer. *Arch Gen Psych,* **38**, 527-533.

Stavraky, KM(1968). Psychological factors in the outcome of human cancer. *J Psychosom Res,* **12**, 251-259.

Stedeford, A (1981a). Couples facing death. I. Psychosocial aspects. *Br Med J,* **ii**, 1033-1036.

Stedeford, A (1981b). Couples facing death. II. Unsatisfactory communication. *Br Med J,* **ii**, 1098-1101.

Stedeford, A (1984). *Facing Death: Patients, Families and Professionals.* Heinemann: London.

Steinburg, MD, Juliano, MA and Wise, L (1985). Psychological outcome of lumpectomy versus mastectomy in the treatment of breast cancer. *Am J Psychiatry,* **142**, 34-39.

Stoll, BA (Ed) (1979). *Mind and Cancer Prognosis.* Wiley: Chichester.

Storr, A (1979). *The Art of Psychotherapy.* Secker & Warburg/Heinemann Medical: London.

Sugarbaker, PH, Barofsky, I, Rosenberg, SA and Gianola, FJ (1981). Quality of life assessment of patients in extremity sarcoma clinical trials. *Surgery,* **91**, 17-23.

Taylor, SE (1983). Adjustment to threatening events. *Am Psychol,* November, 1161-1173.

Thomas, CB, Duszynski, KR and Shaffer, JW (1979). Family attitudes reported in youth as potential predictors of cancer. *Psychosom Med,* **41**, 287-301.

Twycross, RG and Guppy, D (1985). Prednisolone in terminal breast and bronchogenic cancer. *Practitioner,* **229**, Oc27,7057-59.

Waters, WE, Nichols, S, Wheeller, MJ, Fraser, JD and Hayes, AJ (1983). Evaluation of a health education campaign to reduce the delay in women presenting with breast symptoms. *Community Med,* **5**, 104-104.

Watson, M (1983). Psychosocial intervention with cancer patients: a review. *Psychol Med,* **13**, 839-846.

Weisman, AD and Worden, JW (1975). Psychosocial analysis of cancer deaths. *Omega,* **6**, 61-75.

Whitlock, FA and Siskind, M (1979). Depression and cancer: a follow-up study. *Psychol Med,* **9**, 747-752.

Williams, C (1983). *All About Cancer.* Wiley: Chichester.

Wing, JK, Cooper, JE and Sartorius, N (1974). *Measurement and Classification of Psychiatric Symptoms.* Cambridge University Press: Cambridge.

Zigmond, AS and Snaith, RP (1983). The Hospital Anxiety and Depression Scale. *Acta Psychiatr Scand,* **67**, 361-370.

# Index

Acceptance of cancer diagnosis, 43, 72, 83, 107
Adjuvant treatments, 60, 61, 65–67
Alcoholism, 57
'Alternative therapy', 96, 126, 127
Amitriptyline, 91
Amputation, 59
Androgens, 69
Animal experiments, 6
Anger, 24, 28, 45, 47, 114, 116
Antidepressant drugs, 91–92, 114
Anxiety
  and cancer phobia, 40–41
  and chemotherapy, 64
  and delay in presentation, 35–38
  and depression, 82
  and diagnosis of cancer, 44, 47
  and screening, 34
  and survival time, 124, 126
  in long term survivors, 119
  in relatives, 100, 102, 103
Attitudes to cancer, 70–75, 123–124, 125–126

Behaviour patterns and cancer, 30–31
Bereavement
  as precursor of cancer, 9–18
  features of, 115–118
Bowel cancer, 20, 31, 33
  *see also* Colostomy

Brain
  organic brain syndromes, 90–91, 107
  radiotherapy to, 63
  *see also* Cerebral metastases, *and* Cognitive impairment
Breast cancer
  and coping style, 72–73, 74–75
  and childbearing, 31
  chemotherapy for, 66
  delay in presentation, 36–37
  depression preceding diagnosis, 20–21
  depression following diagnosis, 86
  doctor–patient communication, 80
  life events preceding diagnosis, 13–14, 15–18
  hormone treatment, 69
  personality and, 28
  prognosis of, 123–124, 125, 126
  screening for, 32
  social function and, 120
  surgery for, 58
  *see also* Mastectomy
Breast self-examination, 32

Carcinoma, 3
Cerebral metastases, 19, 84, 113
Cervix, cancer of (Cervical cancer), 27–28, 31, 63
Chemotherapy, 64–69
Childhood cancer, 14, 63, 65, 102–103, 116–118, 120

Cigarettes, 30
Cognitive impairment, 64
　see also Organic brain syndromes
Cognitive therapy, 92
Colostomy, 56
　see also Bowel cancer
Communication
　with doctors, 45–47, 57–58, 76–81, 110–112
　within families, 101, 102, 115
Continuing care units, 107–115
Control subjects in research, 7–8, 11
Coping style, 70–75
　see also Attitudes to cancer
Cortisone, 126
Counselling, 58, 94–98
Curative treatment, 51, 65
Cured patients, 119–120
Cushingoid appearance, 69
Cytotoxic drugs, see Chemotherapy

Death, see Bereavement, and Terminal cancer
Delay
　in presentation, 35–39
　in treatment, 38–39, 45
Delusions, 41
Denial, 73–74
　and communication problems, 76–77, 79, 115
　and delay, 35, 37–38
　and counselling, 95
　and diagnosis, 43, 47
　and prognosis, 123
　in relatives, 114
　misuse of term, 56
Depression, 82–93
　and bereavement, 116
　and cancer phobia, 40–41
　and chemotherapy, 64, 66, 67
　and colostomy, 56
　and counselling, 96
　and diagnosis of cancer, 44, 47
　causes of, 84–85
　diagnostic criteria, 83–84
　frequency of, 85–87
　helplessness and, 73
　in relatives, 100, 103
　mastectomy and, 54
　preceding cancer, 10, 19–23, 25　prognosis and, 124
　steroids and, 69
　symptoms of, 82–83
　terminal cancer and, 113–114
　treatment of, 90–93
Dexamethasone, 69
Doctors
　attitudes and behaviour, 38, 77, 90, 111–112
　doctor–patient communication, 45–47, 57–58, 76–81, 110–112
　see also GPs
Dormancy of cancer, 122

Effort after meaning, 11, 14
Elation, 69
Electroconvulsive therapy (ECT), 92–93
Euthanasia, 113

Family, 99–104, 114–115
Fear, 35, 36
Fighting spirit, 73, 109, 123, 125
Followup clinics, 81, 119

General practitioners (GPs), 36, 78, 94
　see also Doctors
Grief, 115–118
　see also Bereavement

Group counselling, 95, 96, 97, 103
Guilt
　and bereavement, 116
　and diagnosis of cancer, 44, 47, 119
　and prognosis, 124
　as precursor of cancer, 10, 12

HAD scale, 84, 113
Hallucinations, 41
Health education, 36, 37
Helplessness/hopelessness, 27, 72, 123, 124
Hodgkin's disease, 65, 78
Hormones
　and cancer growth, 19, 122, 125
　in treatment, 69
Hospices, 107–115
Hostility, 24, 123, 124, 125
Hypochondriasis, 40–42, 116

Ignorance, 35, 36, 47
Imipramine, 91
Immunity, 4, 9, 122, 123, 126
Implants, radioactive, 60
Infertility, 63
Initiating factors, 6

Laryngectomy, 57
Latent period, 7, 8, 9
Leukaemia
　chemotherapy for, 65
　definition, 4
　families of patients, 103, 116–117, 120
　life events preceding, 15
　survival from, 63
Life events
　and depression, 22, 87
　and prognosis of cancer, 122, 125
　as precursors of cancer, 9–18, 19
　definition, 10
Longterm survival, 119–120, 123
Lumpectomy, 58, 60
Lung cancer
　chemotherapy for, 67–68
　depression after diagnosis, 86–90
　depression before diagnosis, 21–22
　doctor–patient communication in, 78–80
　life events preceding diagnosis, 15
　personality in, 26–27
　radiotherapy for, 62–63
　reaction to diagnosis, 46–47
　surgery for, 57
Lymphoma
　chemotherapy for, 65
　definition, 4
　depression after diagnosis, 86
　doctor–patient communication, 78
　survival after, 63

Mammography, 32
Marriage, 100–101, 102, 115
Mastectomy, 54–56, 58–59
　*see also* Breast cancer
Mastery, 75, 126
Meditation, 126–127
Melanoma, 124
Mental defence mechanisms (ego defences), 37, 48
Metastases, 4, 19
　*see also* Cerebral metasteses
Mianserin, 91
MMPI, 25, 28
Monoamine oxidase inhibitors (MAOIs), 91

Nurses, 111–112
Nurse-counsellors 58, 94

Oestrogens, 69
Organic brain syndromes, 90–91, 107

Palliative treatment, 51, 60, 61, 67–68, 108
Pancreas, cancer of, 20
Parents of children with cancer, 102–103, 116–118, 120
Passivity, 122, 123
Personality
   and predisposition to cancer, 24–29, 30
   and reaction to cancer, 43, 70, 76, 84, 109
Phenelzine, 91
Phobias of cancer, 40–42
Pill, contraceptive, 31
Plastic surgery to breast, 58
Prednisolone, 69
Present state examination, 103
Prognosis of cancer, and psychological factors, 121–128
Promoting factors, 6
Prospective studies, 7
Prostate, cancer of, 69
Psychiatrist, referral to, 58, 93
Psychotherapy, 92
   see also Counselling

Radical treatment, 51, 60, 61
   see also Curative treatment
Radiotherapy, 58, 60–63
Rationalization, 56
Relatives, 99–104, 114–115
Religion, 43, 70, 110, 117
Retrospective studies, 7–8

Sarcoma, 3–4, 59
Schizophrenia, 41
Screening
   for cancer, 32–34
   for mood disorder, 84
Self-esteem, 82, 83
Self-help groups, 95, 103
Sexual problems
   and cervical cancer, 63
   and colostomy, 56
   and mastectomy, 54, 55
Side effects
   of chemotherapy, 64–67
   of radiotherapy, 60–61
Skin cancer, 31
   see also Melanoma
Smoking, 30
Social difficulties, 84, 125
Social work, 95, 103
Staff caring for terminal patients attitudes, 117
   selection and support, 112
   see also Doctors
Steroids, 69
Stigma, 44, 119–120
Stoic acceptance, 72, 123
Suicide, 48, 57, 82, 85
Suppression, 37
Surgery, 53–59

Tamoxifen, 69
Terminal cancer, 107–115
Testicular tumours, 65, 123
Tricyclic drugs, 91–92
Twin studies, 15

Unemployment, 56, 120

Widowhood, 11–12, 114, 125